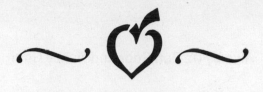

# Eater's Choice
# Low-Fat Cookbook

## Also by Dr. Ron Goor and Nancy Goor

*Eater's Choice: A Food Lover's Guide to
Lower Cholesterol*

*Choose to Lose: A Food Lover's Guide to
Permanent Weight Loss*

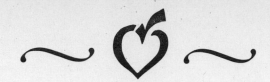

# Eater's Choice
# Low-Fat Cookbook

## Eat Your Way to Thinness
## and Good Health

Dr. Ron Goor and Nancy Goor

Illustrations by Nancy Goor

HOUGHTON MIFFLIN COMPANY
Boston   New York
1999

*Library of Congress Cataloging-in-Publication Data*

Goor, Ron.
Eater's choice low-fat cookbook : eat your way to thinness
and good health / Ron Goor and Nancy Goor.
p.    cm.
Includes index.
ISBN 0-395-97104-7
1. Low-fat diet — Recipes.    I. Goor, Nancy.    II. Title.
RM237.7.G663    1999
641.5'638 — dc21    99-18147  CIP

Some of the recipes in this book previously appeared in
*Eater's Choice* by Dr. Ron Goor and Nancy Goor

Printed in the United States of America

QUM 10 9 8 7 6 5 4 3 2

In loving memory of Helen Miller,
who was a wonderful mother and a wonderful cook

And to Suzanne Lieblich,
a wonderful friend
who has greatly enhanced this book
with many of her scrumptious recipes

# Acknowledgments

The authors wish to thank Mary Evelyn Bedenbaugh, Sharon Bergner, Buffie Brownstein, Letitia Cornelius, Karen Feinstein, Leslie Goodman-Malamuth, Alex Goor, Dan Goor, Jeanette Goor, Lisa Eisen, Anita Hamel, Barbara Hilberg, Eleanor Iversen, Sally and Carl Jones, Ann Jons, Esther Krashes, Suzanne Lieblich, Eva MacLowry, Don Mauer, Helen Miller, Ted Mummery, Dr. James and Ruth Phang, Lona Piatigorsky, Muriel Rabin, Lian Tsao, Philip Wagenaar, Paula Wickstrom, and Linda York.

# Contents

# Introduction

*Eater's Choice Low-Fat Cookbook* is both a new and an old member of Ron and Nancy Goor's family of healthy eating books. Nine years ago, 200 of these recipes formed the Cook's Choice section of the newly published *Eater's Choice: A Food Lover's Guide to Lower Cholesterol*. Over the years the number of recipes grew until *Eater's Choice* contained 290 recipes. The book became so huge (631 pages) — readers would lift it if they misplaced their weights — that the Goors decided to put the recipes in a separate low-fat cookbook. This change has an added benefit: the cookbook is not limited to people with concerns about cholesterol; everyone interested in cooking low-fat food now has a wonderful collection of recipes.

The original recipes were developed when, at age thirty-one, Ron learned that his cholesterol was 311 mg/dl (super-high) and that he could lower it by changing his diet. Nancy Goor didn't want to eat boiled chicken and Jell-O, so she developed the tasty low-sat-fat recipes that the Goors, their two sons, other family members, and guests ate happily. These recipes became Cook's Choice. Each new edition of *Eater's Choice* incorporated more new Goor-tested recipes. When the Goors wrote *Choose to Lose,* they realized the impact of total fat on weight loss and health. Nancy set about reducing the fat in many of the recipes and creating new ones that were much lower in fat.

In this edition, Nancy has added fifty-three great new recipes. Asparagus Soup, Garlicky Potato Soup, Orange Chicken Chinoise, Suzanne's Chickenburgers, Jambalaya, Salmon Sublime, Sweet and Sour Shrimp, Lisa's Vegetable Stew, Multi-Grain Bread, Special Vegetable Salad, Tangy Salad Dressing, Lemon Cheesecake, and Cocoa Meringue Kisses are just a few. She has made improvements on some of the original recipes, culled some of the old ones, and made the number of servings more practical in others. She has completely modified the desserts so that most are very low in fat.

When *Eater's Choice* was first written, reducing saturated fat was the aim; all of the recipes in the book were low-low in saturated fat. However, in the 1995 edition quite a few of the dessert recipes were still high in total fat. For the *Eater's Choice Low-Fat Cookbook,* Nancy wanted all of the recipes to be truly low in fat. She experimented with replacing the fat in cake recipes with applesauce. Yes, applesauce. She was skeptical at first but found that the margarine or oil in a cake recipe could be replaced with applesauce and the results were still delicious.

As you can see, the Goors' books are always evolving and changing with the needs of the times.

*Eater's Choice Low-Fat Cookbook* is still a perfect companion to *Choose to Lose* and *Eater's Choice.* People following either book (as well as anyone else who wants to lose weight and/or lower cholesterol) need recipes that will make them content and satisfied as well as healthy and lean. *Eater's Choice Low-Fat Cookbook* fills the bill. In addition, the recipes are generally quick and easy to make. Nancy Goor loves to eat, but she doesn't like to spend a lot of time in the kitchen.

The Goors wrote *Eater's Choice* to show people that eating healthfully can be a pleasure. They offer you this wish: "We hope you enjoy these recipes as much as we do!"

## A NOTE ON THE RECIPES

You may wonder why we include no red meat and almost no cheese in the recipes. Of course, people may fit beef or cheese into their diets, but we feel that including them in the book would be equating them with healthy food, and we don't consider them healthy. Except for the desserts, all of the recipes in *Eater's Choice Low-Fat Cookbook* may be eaten on a daily basis. If people eat only the recipes in this book (again except for the desserts), they will attain a healthy weight and maintain it forever.

*Be advised:* Because the Goors' oven may not be calibrated with your oven, and your chicken breasts or swordfish steaks may be thicker or thinner than ours, consider the baking time in recipes an estimate. If the recipes tells you to bake a dish for 45 minutes, check your oven at 30 minutes. Your food may be ready.

## HINTS FOR QUICK AND EASY MEAL MAKING

Preparing dinner need not be a three-hour endeavor. If you plan ahead, meal making can be quick and easy. Here are some hints:

- At the beginning of the week, glance through *Eater's Choice Low-Fat Cookbook* or other low-fat cookbooks and choose recipes for the week. Jot down the ingredients you will need so you won't waste time when you shop. Be sure to add foods such as fruits, vegetables, and bread, which you will need for snacks, side dishes, and desserts.
- When you go to the supermarket, follow your shopping list, but if you see a food that entices you, buy it. For example, perhaps you hadn't thought of making Shrimp Creole, but the shrimp look so large and appetizing, you decide to buy them for that night's dinner.
- Buy enough food so you have plenty of material to work with. Buy a variety of vegetables so you can always have one or two with dinner. Make sure you keep your larder (excuse the expression) well stocked with the basics (see Stocking Up, page xv).
- Cook several soups (double or triple the recipes) over the weekend. Freeze them in small containers (enough for one meal) to reheat and eat through the week.
- Make enough of an entrée so you can eat it for two days. Make even more so you can freeze some to reheat later.
- To save preparation time, flour chicken breasts and bake them (with no fat) the night before so you can use them in a recipe the next day.
- Make enough rice for several days. Each day, add a little water and heat up enough for that meal.
- Try basmati rice. It cooks in ten minutes and has a delicious flavor.
- Store canned chicken broth in the refrigerator. The cold hardens the fat so you can remove it easily.

## FOR SUPERIOR TASTE

- Use freshly ground black pepper. There really is a difference between the stale, tasteless pepper that comes in a can and flavorful pepper that has just been ground. It is definitely worth buying a peppermill (usually not expensive) and whole peppercorns (available in the spice section of your grocery store).
- When a recipe calls for nutmeg, grate a whole nutmeg (available in the spice section of your grocery store) for a fresher, nuttier taste.
- Fresh garlic, available in the produce section of your grocery store, is far superior in flavor to garlic powder or garlic salt. It will stay fresh for weeks in the refrigerator.
- Fresh ginger root, available at many grocery stores, can be kept for months in the refrigerator in a jar filled with sherry. Slice off the outer covering and use chopped or grated ginger root for superior results in recipes that call for ginger (but not in cake or cookie recipes).
- Use a zester to intensify the flavor of lemon, lime, or orange peel.

## FAT-REDUCING COOKING EQUIPMENT

- Cast iron makes a great nontoxic, nonstick cooking surface. You can purchase cast-iron griddles that fit over two stove burners and quickly cook chicken breasts, turkey cutlets, French toast, and pancakes with little or no added fat. Smaller cast-iron griddles that fit over one stove burner are also available.
- A steamer cooks vegetables with no fat. Put an inexpensive metal steamer in a saucepan filled with about an inch of water. Place cut-up fresh vegetables on the open "leaves," cover the saucepan, and steam the vegetables until they are tender. For added flavor, mix in some pressed garlic, vinegar, or herbs (thyme, basil, etc.) or top cooked vegetables with a dollop of nonfat yogurt mixed with Dijon mustard.
- A clay cooker keeps chicken moist and tender in the oven without adding fat.
- A gravy skimmer removes fat from canned chicken broth.

## OUR FAVORITE COOKING GADGETS

- Defrosting tray: If you are like Nancy Goor and sometimes forget to thaw chicken breasts in time for preparing dinner, the defrosting tray (one brand is called Miracle Thaw) is a lifesaver. Just run the black metal sheet under hot water until it becomes hot, place the frozen breasts on it, and fifteen minutes later you will have almost or completely thawed meat. If the meat is not completely thawed, repeat the process. Buying the defrosting tray was Ron's idea. Nancy was skeptical until she tried it.
- Vegetable peeler: Good Grips makes the best vegetable peeler in the world. It works like a dream.
- Lemon zester: What a neat gadget! Just press the zester as you pull it down a lemon and you create skinny, fragrant pieces of lemon zest.
- Garlic press: The easiest way to mince garlic for most recipes is just to squeeze it through a garlic press.
- Mini-chopper: You may have noticed how many of our recipes use garlic and ginger. A mini-chopper makes mincing cloves of garlic and ginger root effortless. If you have no lemon zester, you can chop strips of lemon peel (just the yellow) and create grated lemon zest.
- Tea strainer: Use a tea strainer (pictured below) to skim the fat from canned chicken broth.

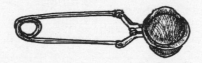

## STOCKING UP

Here is a list of foods and spices to keep in your cupboard, freezer, and refrigerator so you will always have the ingredients you need to create phenomenal meals.

### Foods to Keep on Your Shelves

almonds, slivered

anchovies

apricot jelly

apricots, dried

artichoke hearts in water

baking powder

baking soda

barley

beans, dried (black, pink, etc.)

beans, kidney, canned

chicken broth

chickpeas

cocoa, unsweetened

cornstarch

cream of tartar

flour, unbleached white

flour, whole-wheat

honey

lentils

molasses

oat bran

oatmeal (not quick-cooking)

olive oil

olives, black and green

pasta (spaghetti, noodles, etc.)

peaches, canned

peanuts, unsalted

pineapple chunks, canned

prunes

raisins

salt

sherry, dry

sugar, brown

sugar, confectioners'

sugar, white

tomatoes, canned

tomato juice

tomato paste

tomato sauce

vanilla

vermouth

vinegar

yeast (if you plan to make bread)

### Asian Foods to Keep on Your Shelves

bamboo shoots, canned

bean sauce

black beans (fermented)

chili paste with garlic

hoisin sauce

sesame chili oil

sesame oil

soy sauce and double black soy sauce

water chestnuts, canned

## Spices and Herbs

basil leaves
caraway seeds
cardamom, ground
cayenne pepper
chili powder, hot (if you like)
chili powder, mild
cinnamon, ground
cinnamon sticks
cloves, ground and whole
coriander
cumin, ground and seeds
curry powder

dillweed
ginger, ground
mustard seed, black
nutmeg, whole
oregano
paprika
peppercorns, black
rosemary leaves
sesame seeds
tarragon
thyme leaves
turmeric

## Foods to Keep in Your Freezer

chicken breasts, boneless and
   skinless
corn, frozen
margarine

peas, frozen
turkey cutlets
whole-wheat bread
whole-wheat pita bread

## Foods to Keep in Your Refrigerator

buttermilk
ginger root (store in jar with
   sherry)
margarine

mayonnaise or salad
   dressing
mustard, Dijon
yogurt, nonfat plain

## All-Season Foods to Keep on Hand

carrots
celery
garlic, fresh
lemons
limes
onions
peppers, green

potatoes, sweet
potatoes, white
spinach
squash (acorn, butternut, etc.)
tomatoes
zucchini

# Eater's Choice
# Low-Fat Cookbook

# ~1~
# Soups

**SOUP! WHAT A WONDERFUL INVENTION!** Hot, cold, spicy, sweet, thick, thin, bland, tart — an unlimited source of goodness. Soup is the perfect way to start a meal. It is a delight to the senses and is filling. In fact, a bowl of soup makes you feel so satisfied that by the time you get to the main course, your ravenous hunger has abated and you may eat less for the rest of the meal.

These are the major advantages of making your own soup:

- It will taste much better than anything you can buy.
- You have an enormous choice of great soups to make.
- You need not worry about whether the soup is too salty or fatty because you control the amount of salt and fat.
- You make the kind of soup you want when you want it: hot soup to warm you in the winter, cold soup to refresh you in the summer.
- You can make a large amount at one time and freeze it in small containers for use at a later time. Frozen soup is like money in the bank.

TIP: Store canned chicken broth in the refrigerator. The cold hardens the fat so it is easy to remove.

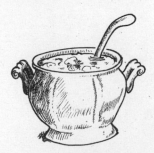

## CHICKEN STOCK

Instead of using canned chicken broth, you can make your own chicken stock and freeze it in small amounts. It will be tastier and will have no fat or salt. There are many ways to make chicken stock; here is one example.

4 pounds chicken backs, or a 4–
   5 pound stewing chicken, or
   6–8 boneless chicken breasts
1 onion, sliced
2 carrots, cut into thirds
1 stalk celery, cut into thirds

1 bay leaf
2 sprigs parsley
¼ teaspoon thyme
1 can (10¾ oz) chicken broth,
   strained

In your largest kettle, combine all ingredients, cover with water, and bring to a boil. Reduce heat, cover, and simmer for 1½ hours.

Remove chicken and vegetables. (You may save both the chicken and the vegetables for another use.)

Refrigerate stock in kettle overnight.

Skim off fat.

Freeze in storage containers.

# ASPARAGUS SOUP CHEZ GOOR

Asparagus Soup is simply delicious. We say "simply" because it couldn't be simpler and "delicious" because it tastes so good. You can use more or less of any ingredient and the soup will still be a success.

3 pounds fresh asparagus
2 medium potatoes, cut into
  ½-inch cubes (about 1½ cups)
3 green onions, sliced
3 cans (10¾ oz each) chicken
  broth, defatted
Freshly ground black pepper to
  taste
½–¾ cup nonfat yogurt

Snap off the stalk ends of the asparagus and discard. Wash asparagus well.

Cut off asparagus tips and place in small saucepan. Cover with water. Set aside.

Cut stalks into 1-inch pieces.

Place asparagus, potatoes, and green onions in a large soup pot. Add broth to cover. Add pepper to taste.

Bring soup to a boil. Lower heat and simmer for about 10 minutes or until asparagus and potatoes are tender.

Meanwhile, bring asparagus tips to a boil, then simmer for 1–3 minutes, until tender but crisp. Set aside.

In a blender, purée soup mixture until smooth. Add yogurt and blend. Add asparagus tips and serve.

*9 one-cup servings (approximately)*
*Calories per serving: 77 total; 0 fat; 0 sat-fat*

# AVGOLEMONO SOUP
## (Greek Lemon Soup)

Avgolemono Soup is both elegant and soothing. It is quick, easy to prepare, and delicious.

½ cup long-grain rice
2 quarts chicken stock, or 3 cans
 (10¾ oz each) chicken broth,
 defatted, + 3 cans water
1½ cups spaghetti broken into
 1-inch pieces

1 egg
1 egg white
Juice of 1½ lemons

In a soup pot, bring stock to a boil, reduce heat, cover, and simmer with rice until tender (about 20 minutes).

Add spaghetti pieces and simmer for the time specified on the spaghetti package.

Just before serving, beat together egg and egg white.

Slowly add lemon juice to the eggs, beating constantly.

Take 1 cup of broth from the soup pot and add it to the lemon-egg mixture, beating constantly.

Pour lemon-egg broth back into the soup pot, beating constantly. Bring to a boil and serve immediately.

*9 one-cup servings*
*Calories per serving: 99 total; 6 fat; 2 sat-fat*

# BARLEY-VEGETABLE SOUP

A hearty soup that improves as it ages. Make it in the morning or the night before so it will have time to thicken.

½ cup pearl barley
2 quarts homemade chicken
   stock, or 3 cans (10¾ oz each)
   chicken broth, defatted,
   + 3 cans water
1 small onion, cut into fourths
1 carrot, cut into thirds
1 stalk celery, cut into 1-inch
   slices

1 teaspoon thyme
1 bay leaf
Freshly ground black pepper to
   taste
3–5 carrots, sliced
2 stalks celery, sliced
½ zucchini, sliced
½ cup onion, chopped
2 cups fresh spinach, chopped

Place barley, chicken stock, onion quarters, carrot thirds, celery slices, thyme, bay leaf, and pepper in a large soup pot and bring to a boil. Reduce heat, cover, and simmer for about 1 hour or until barley is tender.

Add sliced carrots, celery, zucchini, and chopped onion and cook until tender.

Add spinach a few minutes before serving.

*9 one-cup servings*
*Calories per serving: 100 total; 0 fat; 0 sat-fat*

# Bean Soups

Even if you don't like beans, you'll love the following bean recipes: the secret to great bean soup is making a purée of most of the beans instead of leaving them whole. (Of course, you may prefer your beans not puréed at all.)

## BEAN SOUP WITH SPINACH, SQUASH, AND TOMATOES

2 cups dried red chili beans (or any other dried bean)

1 can chicken broth (10¾ oz), defatted

1 medium onion, minced

3 cloves garlic, minced

1 teaspoon minced ginger root

1 teaspoon olive oil

¾–1 teaspoon cumin

¾–1 teaspoon turmeric

½ teaspoon coriander

¼–½ teaspoon cayenne pepper

1 medium zucchini, quartered and sliced into ½-inch pieces

5 ounces fresh spinach, torn into bite-size pieces

1 can (16 oz) chopped tomatoes, with juice

1 cup water

Cover beans with boiling water and let soak for 4 hours. Drain. Add water to cover and cook 1 hour or until tender. Drain.

Remove about ⅞ of the beans and purée with chicken broth in blender. Add purée back to the whole beans. Set aside.

In a large soup pot, sauté onion, garlic, and ginger root in olive oil. Add a splash of water and cook vegetables until soft.

Mix in cumin, turmeric, coriander, and cayenne.

Stir in bean mixture, zucchini, and spinach.

Add tomatoes. If mixture is too thick, slowly add water, a few tablespoons at a time, until desired consistency is reached. Cook 5 minutes.

*10 one-cup servings*
*Calories per serving: 154 total; 8 fat; 0 sat-fat*

# GREAT BLACK BEAN SOUP

1½ cups dried black beans
4 carrots, sliced
1 clove garlic, minced
½ cup chopped onion
1 teaspoon olive oil
1 tablespoon cumin
1 teaspoon coriander

¼–½ teaspoon cayenne
2 cans chicken broth (10¾ oz each), defatted
½ cup long-grain rice
1 cup water
2 tablespoons nonfat yogurt per serving

Cover beans with boiling water. Let soak for 4 hours. Cook them for 1–1¼ hours or until tender. Set aside.

Steam carrots until tender. Set aside.

In a large soup pot, sauté garlic and onion in olive oil. Add a splash of water to help vegetables cook.

Stir in cumin, coriander, and cayenne, and cook briefly. Add chicken broth.

Drain beans and add them to the soup. Add all but 1 cup of carrots. Simmer for 5 minutes. Add rice and simmer, partially covered, for 15–20 minutes.

Purée ¾–⅞ of the soup in blender. Return purée to pot. Add remaining carrots.

If soup is too thick, add water a little at a time until soup is a desirable consistency — not too thick and not too watery.

Top with a dollop of yogurt (2 tablespoons) for each serving.

*7 one-cup servings*
*Calories per serving: 227 total; 11 fat; 1 sat-fat*

## SWEET CABBAGE SOUP

4 cups chopped cabbage
3 cups grated carrot
1 large can (28 oz) tomatoes
    with juice
1 teaspoon tarragon

1 teaspoon basil
1 teaspoon salt (optional)
Water
Juice of 1 lemon
¼ cup raisins

In a large pot, combine cabbage, carrots, tomatoes and their juice, tarragon, basil, and salt. Add water to cover.

Bring to a boil. Reduce heat, cover, and simmer until vegetables are tender.

Purée soup lightly in blender so it still has texture.

Add lemon juice and raisins.

*9 one-cup servings*
*Calories per serving: 56 total; 1 fat; 0 sat-fat*

## CANTALOUPE SOUP

As well as being just plain delicious, cantaloupe is an excellent source of vitamins A and C and fiber. Combined with ginger, orange juice, and buttermilk, cantaloupe makes a refreshing and unusual summer soup.

2 cantaloupes, chilled if possible
¼ cup orange juice
1 teaspoon chopped ginger root

3 tablespoons sweet vermouth
½ cup buttermilk

Halve melons, discard seeds, scoop out meat, and place it in blender.

Add orange juice, ginger, vermouth, and buttermilk, and blend.

If mixture is cold, serve immediately. Otherwise, chill.

*6 one-cup servings*
*Calories per serving: 80 total; 0 fat; 0 sat-fat*

# CARROT SOUP

Carrot Soup is a great spur-of-the-moment dish because it is simple to make and you probably have the ingredients on hand. It is thick and tasty — wonderful to warm the soul and body on a nippy winter day.

1 medium onion, chopped
3 small cloves garlic, minced
1 teaspoon thyme
12 carrots, sliced (about 6 cups)
4 potatoes, peeled and cubed
  (about 4 cups)

1 bay leaf
Freshly ground black pepper to
  taste
2 cans (10¾ oz each) chicken
  broth, defatted

In a soup pot or large casserole, combine onion, garlic, and thyme.
Mix in carrots, potatoes, bay leaf, and pepper.
Add chicken broth and enough water to cover vegetables.
Bring soup to a boil. Reduce heat, cover, and simmer for 30 minutes.
Remove bay leaf.
Remove 2 cups of carrots and potatoes and set aside.
Purée soup in blender. Pour back into soup pot.
Mix in reserved carrot-potato mixture.

*12 one-cup servings*
*Calories per serving: 69 total; 0 fat; 0 sat-fat*

## CARROT SOUP DES BASQUES

The fennel seeds and cumin combine with the carrots to give this soup a hearty robustness.

¾ teaspoon fennel seeds

2 green onions, sliced

4 cups sliced carrots

3 cups sliced potatoes

1 small onion, minced

2 cans chicken broth (10¾ oz each), defatted

¼ teaspoon marjoram

½ teaspoon cumin

Crush fennel seeds with the back of a spoon and set aside.

Combine green onions, carrots, potatoes, and onion in a soup pot.

Add chicken broth, plus enough water to cover vegetables.

Add fennel, marjoram, and cumin.

Bring to a boil, reduce heat, and simmer for 30 minutes or until vegetables are soft.

Coarsely purée in a blender.

*7 one-cup servings*
*Calories per serving: 87 total; 0 fat; 0 sat-fat*

# GINGER-CARROT SOUP

This soup can be eaten either cold or warm. The lime and ginger give it an interesting flavor.

1 tablespoon minced ginger
   root
2 cloves garlic, minced
½ cup chopped onion
1 teaspoon olive oil
5 cups sliced carrots

2 cans (10¾ oz each) chicken
   broth, defatted, + 1 can
   water
¼ cup fresh lime juice
   (approximately)
Nonfat yogurt, for garnish

In a soup pot or large casserole, sauté ginger, garlic, and onion in olive oil. Add a splash of water and cook vegetables until tender.

Stir in carrots.

Add chicken broth and water and simmer until carrots are tender (about 20 minutes).

Add lime juice and purée soup in blender until smooth.

Chill or serve warm. Top each soup bowl with a large dollop of yogurt. Do not mix the yogurt into the soup. For a wonderful combination of tastes and textures, take a little bit of yogurt with each spoonful of soup.

*7 one-cup servings*
*Calories per serving: 80 total; 6 fat; 1 sat-fat*

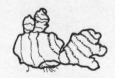

## CAULIFLOWER SOUP

Cauliflower Soup is a treasure. It is simple and quick to make and has a wonderful, delicate taste.

| | |
|---|---|
| 1 large head cauliflower | 1 teaspoon olive oil |
| 1 can chicken broth (10¾ oz), defatted | 2 tablespoons unbleached white flour |
| 2 stalks celery, diced | 1–2 cups water |
| 3 green onions, sliced | |

Remove and discard cauliflower stem. Steam flowerets until tender. Reserve about ½ to 1½ cups and set aside. (You need about 4–5 cups cauliflower for the soup itself. Make sure you don't reserve too much!)

Purée cauliflower and chicken broth in blender. Set aside.

Sauté celery and green onions in oil until tender.

Reduce heat to medium and stir in flour.

Stir in cauliflower purée. Slowly mix in 1 cup of water, stirring constantly until soup thickens. If soup is too thick, stir in remaining water, ¼ cup at a time. Continue cooking until warmed through.

Cut reserved flowerets into bite-size pieces, add to soup, and serve.

*6 one-cup servings (approximately)*
*Calories per serving: 47 total; 7 fat; 1 sat-fat*

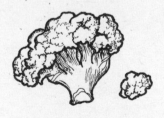

# CORN CHOWDER

1 tablespoon margarine
2 tablespoons flour
2 cups skim milk
2 cans creamed corn (16 oz each)

½ red pepper or green pepper,
chopped

In a large pot, melt margarine.
Remove pot from heat and mix in flour until smooth.
Slowly stir in 1 cup of the skim milk.
Return pot to burner and heat slowly until milk thickens.
Stir creamed corn into milk.
Slowly stir in the remaining 1 cup of skim milk. Heat but do not boil.
Stir in peppers and serve.

*6 one-cup servings*
*Calories per serving: 177 total; 23 fat; 5 sat-fat*

# CUCUMBER SOUP

Cucumber Soup gets a gold star for excellence. It is as refreshing as a dip in a cool lake on a hot summer day. It is simple, quick, and impressive. Be sure to chill the soup thoroughly.

| | |
|---|---|
| 2 cucumbers | 1 clove garlic, crushed |
| 2 cups nonfat yogurt | Walnuts, for garnish |
| 1 can (10¾ oz) chicken broth, defatted | |

Peel cucumbers and cut into bite-size cubes. Salt heavily and set aside.

Spoon yogurt into a medium casserole and stir until smooth.

Stir in chicken broth.

Mix in garlic.

Rinse salt off cucumbers and add them to yogurt mixture. Add salt to taste.

Chill in refrigerator for several hours. Garnish with chopped walnuts.

*5 one-cup servings*
*Calories per serving: 78 total; 0 fat; 0 sat-fat*
*Calories per walnut half: 12 total; 10 fat; 1 sat-fat*

# MONHEGAN ISLAND FISH CHOWDER

Eating Monhegan Island Fish Chowder will show you that fish chowders need not be made with cream to be delicious. This chowder uses one large can of evaporated skim milk, which has 0 calories of fat. A comparable amount of cream has 998 fat calories.

3 large potatoes (about 4 cups)
1 cup chopped onion
1 teaspoon olive oil
2 cups water
1 teaspoon salt (optional)
1 teaspoon basil
¼ teaspoon freshly ground black pepper
1 pound cod fillets
2 cups frozen corn kernels
1 large can (12 oz) evaporated skim milk

Scrub potatoes well and cut into bite-size pieces. *Do not peel.* Steam until just tender. Set aside.

In a large pot, sauté onion in olive oil until tender.

Add potatoes, water, salt, basil, and pepper and bring to a boil. Reduce heat, cover, and simmer for 15 minutes.

Gently place cod fillets on top of potatoes, cover, and simmer until fish flakes easily (about 10 minutes).

Carefully stir in corn and evaporated milk. Heat until corn and milk are hot and serve. Do not allow soup to boil.

*9 one-cup servings*
*Calories per serving: 156 total; 13 fat; 3 sat-fat*

# SUMMER FRUIT SOUP

This is a wonderful, sweet, refreshing soup that couldn't be easier to make. I have made it with blueberries and with strawberries — each makes an elegant and scrumptious soup. To make more or less soup than the recipe calls for, use the same ingredients, just keep the proportions the same.

3 cups strawberries (or other fruit, such as blueberries, raspberries)
2¼ cups water

½ cup sugar
1 cinnamon stick
1–1½ cups nonfat yogurt

Combine fruit, water, sugar, and cinnamon stick in a saucepan.

Bring to a boil and remove from heat. Pour into blender and let cool. (If soup is too hot, it will curdle the yogurt.)

Remove cinnamon stick (but do not discard it) and blend. Add yogurt and blend.

Chill with cinnamon stick. Refrigerate until cold.

*7 one-cup servings*
*Calories per serving: 96 total; 0 fat; 0 sat-fat*

## GAZPACHO I

4 large tomatoes, quartered
1 medium onion, quartered
2 cloves garlic
1 green pepper, quartered
1 cucumber, peeled and quartered

¼ cup white vinegar
1 cup tomato juice
Stale bread (1 or 2 slices, or 1 bagel)

In a blender, roughly purée tomatoes, onion, garlic, green pepper, cucumber, vinegar, and tomato juice. Chill.

Before serving, make croutons by cutting bread (bagel, whole-wheat bread — whatever you have around) into cubes and toasting until crispy in toaster oven.

Garnish soup with croutons.

*8 one-cup servings*

| *Calories per serving:* | *Total* | *Fat* | *Sat-fat* |
|---|---|---|---|
| Without croutons | 55 | 0 | 0 |
| With croutons | 79 | 1 | 1 |

## GAZPACHO II

If you hate wasting the juice from canned tomatoes, this recipe will appeal to you. Each time you use canned tomatoes, accumulate their juice in a storage container in the freezer for future soups.

8 cups juice from canned tomatoes
2 green peppers, quartered
1 medium onion, quartered
2 cloves garlic, minced

1 cucumber, peeled and quartered
¼ cup white vinegar
Salt and freshly ground black pepper to taste

Purée all ingredients in blender. Chill.
Add croutons as in Gazpacho I (above).

*8 one-cup servings*

| *Calories per serving:* | *Total* | *Fat* | *Sat-fat* |
|---|---|---|---|
| Without croutons | 53 | 0 | 0 |
| With croutons | 70 | 1 | 1 |

# HOT AND SOUR SOUP

The ingredients in Hot and Sour Soup seem exotic, but they are all available at Asian food stores. This wonderful soup is worth an extra shopping trip. You may use the ingredients in many other recipes.

NOTE: This soup is spicy hot. Reduce chili oil and white pepper for a milder soup.

10 large dried black
  mushrooms*
½ cup tree ear fungi*
⅓ cup tiger lily stems (golden
  needles)*
2 tablespoons cornstarch
3 tablespoons water
¾ cup diced uncooked chicken
  breast
1 teaspoon olive oil
1 tablespoon soy sauce
1 can (8 oz) bamboo shoots,*
  sliced

6 cups chicken stock, or 3 cans
  (10¾ oz each) chicken broth,
  defatted, + 2 cans water
3 tablespoons white vinegar
1 tablespoon double black soy
  sauce**
2 cakes tofu (fresh bean curd),*
  cubed
2 teaspoons chili oil*
½–1 teaspoon ground white
  pepper
2 egg whites, beaten
4 green onions, sliced

Place mushrooms, tree ears, and tiger lily stems in a small bowl and cover with boiling water. In about 15 minutes or when they are soft, drain off the water and chop off stems or any hard parts.

Slice mushrooms and tree ears and pull tiger lily stems into shreds. Set aside.

Combine cornstarch and water into a smooth paste. Set aside.

In a heated wok or skillet, sauté chicken in oil until chicken is cooked through.

Stir in regular soy sauce.

Stir in mushrooms, tree ears, tiger lily stems, and bamboo shoots.

Add chicken stock, vinegar, and double black soy sauce.

Stir cornstarch mixture into soup. Let thicken.

---

*Available at Asian food stores and some supermarkets.
**If double black soy sauce is not available, make your own by mixing 2 teaspoons regular soy sauce with 1 teaspoon molasses.

Add tofu and bring soup to a boil.

Stir in the chili oil and white pepper.

Turn off the heat for 1 minute and then slowly pour the egg whites into the soup, stirring constantly.

Garnish each bowl of soup with chopped green onions.

*10 one-cup servings*
*Calories per serving: 97 total; 14 fat; 4 sat-fat*

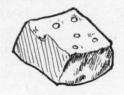

---

### Lentils

Lentils are legumes, which, besides tasting very good, are quite nutritious. They are rich in vitamin C, folic acid, and many minerals. They are a good source of soluble fiber, which has been found to lower blood cholesterol slightly.

---

## LENTIL SOUP

½ pound lentils (1⅓ cups)
½ cup chopped onion
1 cup diced carrots
2 stalks celery, diced
1 green pepper, diced
1 teaspoon olive oil
1 teaspoon cumin
1 teaspoon chili powder
¾ teaspoon allspice

1 bay leaf
¼ cup chopped parsley
1 small boiling potato, peeled
    and diced
1 can chicken broth (10¾ oz),
    defatted
4 cups water
Freshly ground black pepper
½ cup nonfat yogurt

Rinse off lentils and cover with water. Set aside.

In a large soup pot, sauté onion, carrots, celery, and green pepper in olive oil. Add a splash of water and cook vegetables until soft. After about 30 seconds, lower the heat to medium.

Mix in cumin, chili powder, allspice, bay leaf, and parsley.

Drain lentils and add to soup. Mix in potato.

Add chicken broth, water, and pepper.

Bring to boil, cover, and reduce to simmer for about 30 minutes or until lentils are tender.

Remove bay leaf. If you wish, purée about ⅞ of the soup. Return purée to pot and mix into remaining soup.

Serve each bowl with a dollop of yogurt.

*8 one-cup servings*

| *Calories per serving:* | *Total* | *Fat* | *Sat-fat* |
| --- | --- | --- | --- |
| Without yogurt | 141 | 7 | 1 |
| With yogurt | 148 | 7 | 1 |

# LENTIL AND EVERYTHING BUT
# THE KITCHEN SINK SOUP

1 cup lentils

1 clove garlic, minced

2 stalks celery, sliced

½ cup chopped onion

1 teaspoon olive oil

1 cup grated carrot

1½–2 cups coarsely chopped
   potato

5 cups water

1 cup tomato juice

1 teaspoon salt (optional)

1 teaspoon thyme

1 tablespoon soy sauce

⅓ cup brown rice

1½ cups frozen corn

Place lentils in a bowl and cover with water.

In a large pot, sauté garlic, celery, and onion in olive oil. Add a splash of water and cook vegetables until tender.

Stir in carrot and potatoes.

Drain water from lentils and add lentils to vegetables.

Add water, tomato juice, salt, thyme, soy sauce, and brown rice. Bring to a boil. Reduce heat, cover, and simmer until lentils and potatoes are tender (about 30 minutes).

Add corn and cook 10–20 minutes more.

If soup is too thick, add more water, ¼ cup at a time.

*9 one-cup servings*
*Calories per serving: 85 total; 6 fat; 0 sat-fat*

# MINESTRONE

Almost every Italian restaurant in Italy offers its own minestrone, or vegetable soup. Each one is slightly different and all are wonderful. Take whatever vegetables you have in the refrigerator, add some water or broth, pasta, rice and/or beans, to create your own minestrone.

½ onion, sliced

1 teaspoon olive oil

2 potatoes, diced

4 carrots, sliced

2 celery stalks, sliced

¼ cup long-grain rice

1 teaspoon basil

1 teaspoon oregano

½–1 teaspoon salt (optional)

1 can (15½ oz) kidney beans

In a soup pot or large casserole, sauté onion in olive oil. Add a splash of water and continue to cook until tender.

Mix in potatoes, carrots, and celery. Add water to cover.

Add rice, basil, oregano, salt, and kidney beans.

Bring to a boil. Reduce heat, cover, and simmer until rice is cooked and vegetables are tender (about 25 minutes).

*8 one-cup servings*
*Calories per serving: 110 total; 8 fat; 1 sat-fat*

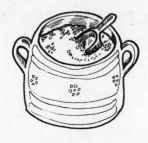

# MULLIGATAWNY SOUP

Customarily, Mulligatawny Soup is made with cream. Our Mulligatawny Soup dispenses with the cream (at 792 fat calories a cup) or a cream substitute. The spicy flavors and interesting textures make this one of our favorite soups.

½ cup chopped onion
½ cup chopped carrot
½ cup chopped celery
2 teaspoons olive oil
1½ tablespoons flour
2 teaspoons curry powder
5 cups chicken stock, or 2 cans
   (10 oz each) chicken broth,
   defatted, + 2 cans water

¼ cup raw long-grain rice
¼ teaspoon thyme
¼ teaspoon freshly ground black
   pepper
½–1 cup diced uncooked chicken
1 apple, peeled and diced

In a soup pot or large casserole, sauté onion, carrot, and celery in oil. Add a splash of water and cook until vegetables are tender.
Stir in flour and curry powder and cook for a few moments.
Pour in chicken stock and bring to a boil.
Add rice, thyme, and pepper and simmer for 15 minutes.
Add chicken and simmer for 5 more minutes.
Add apple and serve.

*6 one-cup servings*
*Calories per serving: 114 total; 14 fat; 2 sat-fat*

## MUSHROOM SOUP

A must! In no more than ten minutes you can make this sophisticated and soothing soup and set it before your family or guests.

½ pound fresh mushrooms, sliced
2 teaspoons olive oil
2 cans (10¾ oz each) chicken broth, defatted

Juice of 1 lemon (about ¼ cup)
2 tablespoons dry vermouth
1 tablespoon dry sherry
Dash of Tabasco sauce

In a medium saucepan, sauté mushrooms in olive oil. Add a splash of water and continue to cook until just tender.

Gently mix in strained chicken broth.

Add lemon juice, vermouth, sherry, and Tabasco sauce, and heat until hot.

*5 one-cup servings*
*Calories per serving: 90 total; 13 fat; 2 sat-fat*

## ORIENTAL NOODLE SOUP

2 cans chicken broth (10¾ oz each), defatted, + 2 cans water
2 ounces cellophane noodles*
1 tablespoon soy sauce

¼ teaspoon white pepper
1 cake tofu,* cubed
1 green onion, sliced
10–15 snow peas

Bring broth and water to a boil in a soup pot. Add cellophane noodles.

Simmer about 10 minutes, until noodles are soft.

Add soy sauce and white pepper. Simmer a minute or two.

Add tofu, green onion, and snow peas and serve.

*6 one-cup servings*
*Calories per serving: 64 total; 8 fat; 1 sat-fat*

---

*Available at Asian food stores and some supermarkets.

# COLD SASSY PEA SOUP

24 oz frozen peas (about 6 cups)
2 cups water
2 cloves garlic, cut in half
2 cups nonfat yogurt
½ cup fresh lime juice (about 4
  limes)

1 teaspoon chili powder
½–1 teaspoon salt (optional)
2–3 teaspoons sliced jalapeño
  pepper, fresh or pickled

### Garnish per bowl

1 tablespoon chopped tomato

1 tablespoon cilantro, chopped

Thaw peas by placing them in a large bowl and adding cold water. Drain water and reserve. You can use this cold water for the 2 cups of water in the recipe.

Place garlic in bottom of blender. Add peas, water, and yogurt and purée until smooth. If you are running out of room in your blender, empty some of the puréed soup into a soup pot or casserole.

Add lime juice, chili powder, salt, and jalapeño peppers and blend until smooth.

Pour into soup pot or casserole and chill until cold.

Garnish with tomato and cilantro.

*9 one-cup servings*
*Calories per serving: 78 total; 2 fat; 0 sat-fat*

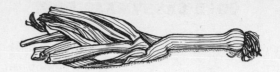

# POTATO SOUP WITH LEEKS AND BROCCOLI

1 tablespoon olive oil
1½ cups sliced leeks* (white part)
2 tablespoons unbleached white
   flour
3½ cups hot water
4 cups peeled and sliced potatoes

1 teaspoon salt (optional)
¼ teaspoon freshly ground black
   pepper
2 cups broccoli flowerets
1½ cups skim milk

In a soup pot, heat olive oil.

Mix in leeks, cover pot, and cook slowly until leeks are soft.

Blend in flour and cook for a few seconds. Remove pot from heat.

Add ½ cup of the hot water and blend thoroughly.

Add the remaining hot water, potatoes, salt, and pepper.

Bring to a boil, reduce heat, and simmer, partially covered, for about 40 minutes or until potatoes are tender.

While the potatoes are cooking, steam the broccoli until it is just tender. Set aside.

Pour the cooked potatoes and their liquid into a blender and purée until they are almost smooth (they should still have some texture).

Return soup to pot, add 1 cup of the skim milk, and blend well.

If the soup is too thick, slowly add more skim milk, ¼ cup at a time. Do not add so much skim milk that the soup becomes too thin. Soup should be *thick*.

Mix in broccoli, correct seasoning, and finish with several twists of your peppermill.

*7 one-cup servings*
*Calories per serving: 113 total; 16 fat; 2 sat-fat*

---

*If you have no leeks, you may use onions, but the special flavor of leeks enhances the soup.

## GARLICKY POTATO SOUP

½ cup chopped onion
1 teaspoon olive oil
8 garlic cloves, chopped fine
7 cups diced potatoes

2 cans (10¾ oz each) chicken
   broth, defatted
½ cup water
1 cup nonfat buttermilk

In a large soup pot, sauté onion in oil until soft.
Mix in garlic and potatoes.
Add broth and water.
Bring to a boil, then simmer until potatoes are tender.
Purée soup in blender and return to pot.
Stir in buttermilk.

*7 one-cup servings (approximately)*
*Calories per serving: 110 total; 5 fat; 0 sat-fat*

## GINGER SQUASH SOUP

½ cup chopped onion
2 tablespoons minced ginger
   root
6 cups butternut squash, peeled,
   seeded, and cut into thin
   slices

2 cans chicken broth (10¾ oz
   each), defatted
4 cloves garlic
2–3 tablespoons fresh lime juice
Salt and freshly ground black
   pepper to taste

In a large soup pot, combine onion, ginger root, and squash.
Add broth and garlic, and bring to a boil.
Reduce heat and simmer, covered, until squash is tender, about 15
minutes.
Purée in blender or food processor.
Return to pot and stir in lime juice, salt, and pepper.
Add more water, a tablespoon at a time, if too thick.

*7 one-cup servings*
*Calories per serving: 52 total; 0 fat; 0 sat-fat*

## SOUR CHERRY SOUP

Sour Cherry Soup is a sweet soup. It is ideal for a luncheon or dinner party and *very* simple to make. It has no fat but does have quite a lot of sugar.

| | |
|---|---|
| 2 cans (1 lb each) undrained sour cherries packed in water | 2 tablespoons unbleached white flour |
| ¾ cup sugar | 6 tablespoons cold water |
| 1 stick cinnamon | 2 cups water |

Remove 12 cherries from one can and put aside for garnish. (Or buy another whole can of cherries.)

In a medium saucepan, cook cherries with their juice, sugar, and cinnamon stick for 10 to 15 minutes.

In a small bowl, mix flour and 3 tablespoons of the cold water until smooth. Blend in remaining 3 tablespoons cold water.

Remove cinnamon stick from cooked cherries and set aside.

Pour cherry mixture into blender. Add flour mixture and blend until soup is smooth.

Return soup to saucepan, add 2 cups water, and heat just to boiling.

Return cinnamon stick to soup and chill.

Garnish each bowl of soup with a few cherries before serving.

*6 one-cup servings*
*Calories per serving: 165 total; 0 fat; 0 sat-fat*

# APPLE-SQUASH SOUP

Apple-Squash Soup is rich and delicious. Use acorn or butternut squash or even summer squash.

2 cups chopped onion
About 3 pounds squash, peeled,
    seeded, and cubed (about
    6 cups)
2 Granny Smith or other tart
    apples, peeled, cored, and
    cubed
3 cups chicken stock, or 1 can
    (10¾ oz) chicken broth,
    defatted, + water to equal
    3 cups

5 teaspoons curry powder
1 cup apple cider or apple juice
Freshly ground black pepper to
    taste
1–2 Granny Smith or other tart
    apples, for garnish

In a large pot, combine onion, squash, apples, and chicken stock. Stir in curry powder. Bring to a boil, reduce heat, and simmer for 25 minutes or until squash and apples are tender.

Remove 2 cups of liquid and set aside.

Purée remaining soup in blender and return to soup pot.

Stir cider into puréed soup.

Add liquid that you set aside, a bit at a time, making sure that soup remains thick, but not *too* thick.

If necessary, reheat soup until hot.

Pepper liberally.

Grate or chop apples into tiny pieces *just* before serving and garnish each bowl of soup.

*9 one-cup servings*
*Calories per serving: 122 total; 0 fat; 0 sat-fat*

# CHILLED STRAWBERRY SOUP

Ron says this soup should be in the dessert section. It is sweet and refreshing and easy to make.

| | |
|---|---|
| 2 oranges, peeled and thinly sliced | 2 cups sliced strawberries* |
| 1 cinnamon stick | Dash of salt |
| 2 cups water | 1½ tablespoons cornstarch |
| ¼ cup sugar | 1 tablespoon water |

Simmer orange pieces and cinnamon stick in 2 cups water for 5 minutes.

Remove the cinnamon stick and set aside.

Add sugar, strawberries, and a dash of salt and bring to a boil. Turn heat to low.

Blend cornstarch with 1 tablespoon water and stir into soup until clear.

Chill with cinnamon stick.

*5 one-cup servings*
*Calories per serving: 90 total; 0 fat; 0 sat-fat*

---

*Try peaches, cherries, apricots, or a combination of fruits.

# COLD TOMATO SOUP

½ teaspoon olive oil
½ cup chopped onion
3 cloves garlic, minced
2 cans (10¾ oz) chicken broth,
   defatted
1 large can (28 oz) tomatoes
½ teaspoon basil

6 black peppercorns
1 bay leaf
½ teaspoon sugar
1 cup nonfat yogurt
4 medium tomatoes, cut into
   bite-size pieces

In a large skillet, sauté onion and garlic in olive oil. Add a splash of water to help cook vegetables.

Add broth, tomatoes with juice, basil, peppercorns, and bay leaf. Heat to boiling and simmer for 10 minutes.

Remove bay leaf and purée soup in blender until smooth.

Let cool for a few minutes.

Add sugar and yogurt and either blend or stir until smooth.

Add cut-up tomatoes. Chill for at least several hours or until very cold.

*9 one-cup servings*
*Calories per serving: 54 total; 2 fat; 0 sat-fat*

## TOMATO-RICE SOUP

If you hate wasting the juice from canned tomatoes, collect it in a storage container in the freezer and save it for Tomato-Rice Soup (also for Gazpacho II). Then, when you have forgotten to plan ahead for soup and have no fresh vegetables in the house, you can raid the freezer for peas, corn, and the juice you have collected. Add some onion, cloves, and rice and *voilà!*

6 cups juice from canned
    tomatoes
1 tablespoon grated onion
1 pinch ground cloves

½ cup long-grain rice
1 cup frozen peas
1 cup frozen corn

Combine tomato juice, onion, cloves, and rice and bring to a boil. Reduce heat and simmer for about 25 minutes.

Add peas and corn.

*8 one-cup servings*
*Calories per serving: 93 total; 0 fat; 0 sat-fat*

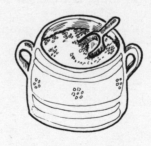

# TORTILLA SOUP

This instantaneous soup always gets rave reviews.

6 corn tortillas*
1 medium onion, diced
3 cloves garlic, minced
1 teaspoon olive oil
2 tablespoons chili powder
1 teaspoon oregano
1 large can (28 oz) heavy
   concentrated crushed
   tomatoes

1 can (10¾ oz) chicken broth,
   defatted, + 1 can water
1 green pepper, diced
1 cup frozen corn
Salt and pepper to taste

About 15 minutes before you serve soup, heat tortillas in a slow oven (325°F), until crisp.

In a soup pot, sauté onion and garlic in oil. Add a splash of water and cook vegetables until soft.

Stir in chili powder and oregano.

Stir in tomatoes, chicken broth, and water.

Bring to a boil and simmer for a few minutes.

Add green pepper and corn.

Add salt and pepper to taste.

For each serving, break a tortilla into small pieces and place at the bottom of a soup bowl. Ladle soup over the tortilla and serve.

*7 one-cup servings*
*Calories per serving: 144 total; 10 fat; 1 sat-fat*

---

*Corn tortillas can be found in the refrigerator section of most supermarkets. Be sure they contain no lard or other saturated fat.

# VEGETABLE SOUP PROVENÇAL

A hearty Mediterranean soup with a distinctive taste. Use whatever vegetables you have on hand. The more the better! The secret ingredient is the pistou. Italy has its pesto and France has its pistou. Both sauces are combinations of basil, garlic, cheese (omitted here because it is high in fat), and olive oil, added to soups and pasta to enhance and enrich the flavor.

Make a lot of Vegetable Soup Provençal. It freezes well.

CAUTION: Reheat slowly.

1 large onion, chopped

3 cups sliced carrots

2–3 potatoes, diced

2½ quarts water

1 teaspoon salt (optional)

Any vegetables, such as:

   1 zucchini, sliced

   2 cups broccoli flowerets

   1 cup cauliflower flowerets

   2 cups green beans

2 slices stale bread, shredded

½ cup broken pieces of spaghetti

### Pistou

8 cloves garlic, minced

⅓ cup chopped parsley

1 can (6 oz) tomato paste

3 tablespoons dried basil, or ½ cup fresh basil

In a large soup pot, combine onion, carrot, and potato.

Add water and salt and heat to boiling. Reduce heat, cover, and simmer for 20 minutes.

Add vegetables, bread, and spaghetti and simmer, covered, for 15 minutes more.

Make pistou in food processor, blender, or with a fork by blending garlic, parsley, tomato paste, and basil until smooth.

Stir the pistou into the soup, a little at a time.

*15 one-cup servings*
*Calories per serving: 58 total; 1 fat; 0 sat-fat*

## VEGETABLE SOUP WITH SPINACH, POTATOES, RICE, AND CORN

This soup is great! So quick, so easy, and so tasty.

2 cloves garlic, minced
1 teaspoon olive oil
10 ounces fresh spinach, torn
   into bite-size pieces
2 cans chicken broth (10¾ oz
   each), defatted, + 4 cans
   water

4 small potatoes, peeled and
   cubed
½ cup long-grain rice
2 cups frozen corn

In soup pot, sauté garlic in oil until soft.
Stir in spinach.
Add broth, water, potatoes, and rice, and bring to a boil.
Reduce to a simmer and cook for about 15 minutes or until potatoes are tender and rice is cooked.
Add corn and cook for about 1 minute.

*10 one-cup servings*
*Calories per serving: 129 total; 12 fat; 2 sat fat*

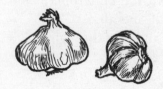

# WATERCRESS SOUP

Watercress Soup is thick and creamy in texture but low in fat. It makes a refreshing first course in summer or winter.

1 teaspoon olive oil
1 cup chopped onion
2 bunches watercress, washed and stems removed
2 tablespoons unbleached white flour
5 cups chicken stock, or 2 cans (10¾ oz each) chicken broth, defatted, + 2 cans water

½ teaspoon freshly ground black pepper
1 teaspoon tarragon
1 teaspoon dillweed
1 quart buttermilk
2 tablespoons fresh lemon juice
1 teaspoon Worcestershire sauce
½ teaspoon curry powder
10 sprigs watercress, for garnish

In a large soup pot, heat olive oil. Add onion and a splash of water and cook until soft.

Stir in watercress.

Cover and cook slowly for 10 minutes or until watercress wilts.

Sprinkle on flour and mix well.

Add chicken stock and pepper. Cover and simmer for 30 minutes. Add tarragon and dillweed at the last minute.

Cool slightly. Purée in blender or food processor.

Return soup to pot. Add buttermilk, lemon juice, and Worcestershire sauce and stir until smooth.

Add curry powder and heat through.

Cool and refrigerate.

*10 one-cup servings*
*Calories per serving: 74 total; 4 fat; 0 sat-fat*

# ZUCCHINI SOUP

One of the greatest recipes known to mankind. Hot or cold, summer or winter, for family or company, Zucchini Soup is delicious — and easy. You can even prepare it 20 minutes before you eat. If you want to make more and freeze it, just add a few more zucchini and more broth. This recipe is very flexible. Add more or less of any ingredient, and it will still taste superb.

3 large or 4 medium zucchini (or
  more or less), sliced
½ cup chopped onion
¼ cup long-grain rice
Chicken stock to cover zucchini,
  or 2 cans (10¾ oz each)
  chicken broth, defatted, +
  water to cover zucchini

1 teaspoon curry powder
  (approximately)
1 teaspoon Dijon mustard
  (approximately)
½–1 cup nonfat yogurt

In a large soup pot, combine zucchini, onion, rice, chicken stock, and water (add more water, if necessary, to cover zucchini).

Simmer for 15 minutes or until zucchini are tender.

Purée in blender, adding curry powder, mustard, and yogurt to taste.

Eat warm or cool.

This soup freezes well. Reheat frozen soup for best results. Eat immediately or cool for later.

*8 one-cup servings (approximately)*
*Calories per serving: 80 total; 0 fat; 0 sat-fat*

## CHUNKY ZUCCHINI VEGETABLE SOUP

A winner!

1 cup chopped onion
1½ cups sliced carrots
2 cloves garlic, minced
1 teaspoon olive oil
¼ cup tomato paste
2 cans (10¾ oz each) chicken
   broth, defatted

3 pounds zucchini, sliced
1–2 teaspoons pickled jalapeño
   pepper (optional)
⅓ cup long-grain rice, uncooked
1 cup water

In a large soup pot, sauté onion, carrots, and garlic in olive oil.
Stir in tomato paste and broth.

Mix in zucchini, pepper, and rice. Add water.

Cover and simmer for 15–20 minutes until rice is cooked and vegetables are tender.

In blender, roughly blend vegetables to an even, chunky consistency. If soup is too thick, add water, ¼ cup at a time.

*9 cups (approximately)*
*Calories per serving: 60 total; 4 fat; 0 sat-fat*

# ~2~
## Chicken

**CHICKEN IS ONE** of the most versatile meats. You can sauté it, bake it, broil it, boil it, roast it, or make it into chicken salad, chicken pot pie, or chicken brochettes. You can cook it with fruit, vegetables, grains, wine, herbs, or spices and it will be different and delicious each time.

Almost all of the following recipes use chicken breasts without skin because they are so versatile. Chicken breast without skin is the preferred choice for anyone concerned about fat intake. A chicken breast without skin contains 13 fat calories. Be sure to remove the skin *before* cooking, as cooking the breast with the skin and then removing it before you eat it raises the fat calories to 28 per breast.

Chicken breasts may be purchased with bones or already boned. You may have avoided buying *boneless* chicken breasts without skin because of their expense. However, the skin and bones of a chicken breast account for half its weight. You are paying much more for chicken breasts with skin and bones than you think. Look for boned chicken breasts without skin on sale for a real bargain.

If chicken breast tenderloins are available in your supermarket, we recommend them highly. They are wonderfully tender. Substitute about 4 tenderloins for 1 chicken breast. Be sure to pull out the tendon.

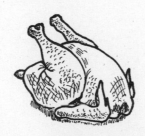

If you use canned chicken broth in any of these recipes, either strain the broth (pour it through a fine tea strainer) or, if the fat is hardened, lift it off the surface of the broth with a spoon. You can also use a gravy skimmer to skim off the fat.

### Saving Sat-Fat and Fat

To save sat-fat and fat calories, flour and bake chicken in a shallow baking pan with no fat instead of sautéing it in oil. When the chicken is fully cooked, either refrigerate or freeze it for later use or substitute it for sautéed chicken in a recipe.

### Cooking for One or Two

If you find that one of our recipes makes more servings than you need, just divide all the ingredients proportionately. For example, if the recipe calls for 8 chicken breasts, use 4 or 2, and instead of ½ cup of lime juice, use ¼ cup or 2 tablespoons; instead of 1 teaspoon of ginger, use ½ teaspoon or ¼ teaspoon, etc. You may also want to make the full or half recipe and eat one half and freeze the rest. If you have a big dinner party, you can double or triple all the ingredients. The recipes are quite flexible, so just relax and adapt them to your needs.

# ALEX'S CHINESE CHICKEN WITH ONIONS, MUSHROOMS, AND ZUCCHINI

1–1½ pounds boneless, skinless
chicken breasts
½ cup unbleached flour
½ teaspoon salt (optional)
¼ teaspoon freshly ground black
pepper
1 medium zucchini
3 tablespoons soy sauce
3 tablespoons white vinegar

1–1½ tablespoons chili paste
with garlic
¼–1 teaspoon red pepper flakes
(optional)
2 tablespoons + 1 cup water
2 tablespoons cornstarch
2 large onions, sliced
1 tablespoon olive oil
3 cups mushrooms, sliced

Preheat oven to 375°F.

Shake chicken in a plastic bag with flour, salt, and pepper until coated. Bake chicken in a single layer in a baking pan until it is cooked through. When chicken is cool enough to handle, cut it into bite-size pieces and set them aside.

Slice zucchini lengthwise into quarters. Cut these into ½-inch pieces. Steam zucchini 1–3 minutes or until tender. Set aside.

Combine soy sauce, vinegar, chili paste, and red pepper flakes and set aside.

Add 2 tablespoons of water to cornstarch and mix until smooth. Add remaining water to cornstarch and set aside.

Sauté onions in the remaining 1 tablespoon olive oil until soft. Add mushrooms and cook for a minute. Stir in chicken.

Add soy sauce and cornstarch mixtures and stir until vegetables and chicken are covered.

Stir in zucchini.

Serve over rice.

*6 generous servings*
*Calories per serving: 192 total; 31 fat; 6 sat-fat*

## CHICKEN WITH APPLES AND ONIONS

6 boneless, skinless chicken
   breasts
1 cup sliced onion
1 teaspoon olive oil

2 cups peeled and sliced apples
1½ cups apple juice
2 tablespoons honey
½–1 teaspoon salt (optional)

Preheat oven to 350°F.

Place chicken breasts in a shallow baking pan.

In a skillet, sauté onions and apples in olive oil. Add a splash of water and cook until tender.

Pour onions and apples over chicken.

In a small saucepan, combine apple juice and honey. Pour over chicken.

Bake for 30–45 minutes or until chicken is cooked through.

This dish tastes good reheated.

*6 servings*
*Calories per serving: 225 total; 20 fat; 1 sat-fat*

# APRICOT CHICKEN DIVINE

One-quarter cup of nonfat yogurt (0 fat calories) replaces ¼ cup of sour cream (108 fat calories) to create this divine chicken.

4 boneless, skinless chicken
   breasts
¼ cup unbleached white flour
½ teaspoon salt (optional)

¼ cup apricot preserves
½ tablespoon Dijon mustard
¼ cup nonfat yogurt
1 tablespoon slivered almonds

Preheat oven to 375°F.

Shake chicken in a plastic bag filled with flour and salt until chicken is coated.

Place chicken in a single layer in a shallow baking pan and bake for 25 minutes.

Combine apricot preserves, mustard, and yogurt.

Spread apricot mixture on chicken and bake for 10–15 minutes more or until done.

Just before serving, brown almonds lightly in toaster oven.

Sprinkle almonds over chicken and serve over rice.

*4 servings*
*Calories per serving: 215 total; 23 fat; 5 sat-fat*

## CHICKEN WITH APRICOTS, PRUNES, AND OLIVES

This dish is colorful to look at and a pleasure to eat. What's more, it is quick and easy and can be prepared ahead of time.

| | |
|---|---|
| 6 boneless, skinless chicken breasts | 3 tablespoons white vinegar |
| ¾ cup dried prunes | ½ cup dry vermouth |
| ½ cup dried apricots | 2 cloves garlic, minced |
| 12 green olives, halved | 2 tablespoons brown sugar |
| 2 teaspoons olive oil | 1 tablespoon oregano |
| | 1 tablespoon capers |

Place chicken breasts in a medium-large bowl or casserole.

Combine prunes, apricots, olives, olive oil, vinegar, vermouth, garlic, brown sugar, oregano, and capers and pour over chicken. Cover and marinate in refrigerator for several hours or overnight.

Preheat oven to 350°F.

Remove chicken from marinade. Arrange in shallow baking pan.

Spread marinade over chicken and bake for 30–45 minutes until chicken is fully cooked.

*6 servings*
*Calories per serving: 256 total; 34 fat; 7 sat-fat*

# GRILLED APRICOT-GINGER CHICKEN

¾ cup dried apricots
Juice of ½ lemon
1 clove garlic, minced
½ teaspoon minced ginger root
¼–½ teaspoon cardamom

⅛–¼ teaspoon cayenne pepper
¼–½ teaspoon salt (optional)
2 teaspoons olive oil
5 boneless, skinless chicken
  breasts

Place apricots in a small saucepan and add water to cover. Add lemon juice, bring to a boil, reduce heat, and simmer until tender.

In a blender or food processor, purée apricots and liquid with garlic, ginger, cardamom, cayenne pepper, salt, and olive oil. Add more water if too thick. Score the chicken breasts several times on each side. Cover with the apricot mixture and marinate in refrigerator for several hours or overnight.

Remove chicken from marinade and reserve marinade.

Preheat oven to broil or prepare grill.

Broil or grill chicken until cooked through.

Heat marinade and spoon over chicken.

Serve over rice.

*5 servings*
*Calories per serving: 191 total; 29 fat; 6 sat-fat*

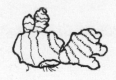

# BAGHDAD CHICKEN

¾ cup chopped onion

2 teaspoons garam masala*

1 teaspoon olive oil

⅓ cup uncooked long-grain rice

⅔ cup water

3 tablespoons raisins

3 tablespoons chopped peanuts

¼ cup nonfat yogurt

8 boneless, skinless chicken breasts

Salt and freshly ground black pepper to taste

4 cups cooked long-grain rice (optional)

Preheat oven to 375°F.

Sauté onion in garam masala and olive oil. Add a splash of water and cook vegetables until soft. Stir in rice.

Add water, cover saucepan, and cook over low heat until liquid is absorbed (about 20 minutes).

Remove from heat. Stir in raisins, peanuts, and yogurt. Let cool.

Flatten chicken breasts between two sheets of wax paper. Salt and pepper chicken.

Put a portion of the rice mixture in the center of each breast.

Bring together the sides of the breast to enclose the rice.

Place the breast seam-side down in a shallow casserole.

Bake until chicken is cooked through (about 30–45 minutes).

Combine any rice mixture you have remaining with plain rice and serve on the side.

*8 servings*
*Calories per serving: 200 total; 38 fat; 7 sat-fat*

---

*Available at specialty food stores. Or make your own by combining ½ teaspoon ground cloves, ¾ teaspoon ground cardamom, and ¾ teaspoon cinnamon.

# BALSAMIC CHICKEN WITH POTATOES AND ONIONS

4 tablespoons balsamic or other
  flavored vinegar
4 boneless, skinless chicken
  breasts
2 medium-large potatoes
¾ cup sliced onion

1 teaspoon olive oil
¼–½ teaspoon thyme
Salt to taste (optional)
Freshly ground black pepper to
  taste

Pour 3 tablespoons of vinegar over chicken and marinate for several hours or overnight.

Preheat oven to 350°F.

Wash potatoes thoroughly and cut into ¼-inch slices. (You should have about 2 cups.) Steam in a vegetable steamer for ten minutes (until almost tender).

Meanwhile, in a small skillet sauté onion in olive oil on medium heat. Add a splash of water and cook vegetables until soft.

Mix in remaining tablespoon vinegar.

Mix in potatoes.

Pour the potato mixture into a shallow casserole large enough to accommodate a layer of potatoes covered by chicken breasts. Sprinkle potatoes with about ¼ teaspoon thyme.

Remove chicken from marinade and place on top of potatoes. Season with salt and pepper to taste and sprinkle with remaining thyme.

Bake for 30–45 minutes or until chicken is cooked through.

*4 servings*
*Calories per serving: 193 total; 23 fat; 5 sat-fat*

## BAR-B-QUE CHICKEN

Bar-B-Que Chicken is a popular main dish with food lovers of all ages. It also makes a great sandwich. Place the barbecued chicken on a slice of bread, top with sauce, a slice of tomato, a few slices of onion, and another slice of bread.

| | |
|---|---|
| 2 tablespoons Dijon mustard | 2 cloves garlic, minced |
| ¼ cup vinegar | Dash of Tabasco sauce |
| ¼ cup molasses | 8 boneless, skinless chicken |
| ½ cup ketchup |     breasts or skinless thighs* |
| ½ teaspoon Worcestershire sauce | |

In a large bowl, mix together Dijon mustard, vinegar, molasses, ketchup, Worcestershire sauce, garlic, and Tabasco for marinade.

Pour about half of the marinade over the chicken and refrigerate the rest to use later.

Marinate chicken for an hour (or less, if you haven't planned ahead).

Remove chicken and reserve marinade.

Barbecue, broil, or use a cast-iron pancake griddle to grill chicken for 10 minutes or until fully cooked.

Turn and coat chicken with marinade and continue cooking until done.

Combine reserved marinade with the marinade you refrigerated. Heat to boiling and simmer for 2 minutes. Spoon over chicken before serving.

*8 servings*

| Calories per serving: | Total | Fat | Sat-fat |
|---|---|---|---|
| 1 breast | 173 | 13 | 4 |
| 1 thigh | 126 | 24 | 6 |

---

*For a barbecue, you may want greater quantities of chicken. Just double, triple, or quadruple the recipe.

# BLACKENED CHICKEN

Ron is in seventh heaven when he bites into a chunk of chicken and the chicken bites back. The spicier it is, the better he likes it. He likes Blackened Chicken a lot.

### Spice Mix

1¼ teaspoons thyme
1¼ teaspoons basil
¾ teaspoon onion powder
¼ teaspoon salt (optional)
½ teaspoon cayenne pepper

¾ teaspoon paprika
¼ teaspoon white pepper
½ teaspoon freshly ground black
    pepper

5 boneless, skinless chicken
    breasts

Combine seasonings on a small plate. Roll each breast in seasonings, coating it on both sides and set it aside on a large plate. For a milder chicken, use less seasoning on each breast.

Either grill on a cast-iron pancake griddle or barbecue, broil, or bake chicken until cooked through. Don't overcook. Top each breast with salsa (page 216).

NOTE: If you are using a cast-iron griddle, don't let it get too hot or it will char the chicken. You may need to turn on your exhaust fan to clear the hot spices from the air.

*5 servings*
*Calories per serving: 130 total; 13 fat; 4 sat-fat*

## SUZANNE'S CHICKENBURGERS

When Estelle Hennefeld's mother passed down her family's Swedish meatball recipe, little did she suppose that her granddaughter Suzanne (whom she never met) would modify the recipe and create these scrumptious low-fat chickenburgers.

The recipe uses 1 pound of boneless, skinless chicken breasts to make 6 burgers, but if you want more, just double, triple, or quadruple the ingredients, keeping the proportion of chicken to vegetables and bread the same.

1 carrot, cut into fourths
1 celery stalk, cut into fourths
½ green or red pepper, cut into fourths
1 small onion, cut into fourths

2 slices whole-wheat bread
1 pound boneless, skinless chicken breasts
Salt to taste

Preheat broiler.

In a food processor, chop the carrot, celery, pepper, and onion to make 2 cups of finely chopped vegetables. Set aside in a small bowl.

Put bread in processor and process to create fine bread crumbs. Set aside in a small bowl.

Cut chicken breasts into quarters and grind in food processor.

In a large bowl, combine ground chicken, vegetables, bread crumbs, and a dash of salt.

Form 6 medium-large patties (or 4–5 very large ones) and place on broiler pan. Broil about 10 minutes or until cooked through. Don't overcook, or the burgers may dry out.

*6 burgers*
*Calories per serving: 98 total; 9 fat; 3 sat-fat*

# CAJUN CHICKEN

8 boneless, skinless chicken
  breasts

½ cup unbleached white flour
½ teaspoon salt, optional

*Seasoning Mix* (Vary amount of peppers for a hotter or milder taste.)

¾ teaspoon oregano
½ teaspoon thyme
½ teaspoon basil
½ teaspoon salt
½ teaspoon paprika

¼ teaspoon freshly ground black
  pepper
½ teaspoon cayenne pepper
¼ teaspoon white pepper

3 cloves garlic, minced
¾ cup chopped onion
2 stalks celery, diced
1 green pepper, chopped
1 tomato, coarsely chopped
1 tablespoon olive oil

1 can (10¾ oz) chicken broth,
  defatted
1 small can (8 oz) tomato sauce
1 potato, peeled and diced
2 bay leaves

Preheat oven to 350°F.

Shake chicken in a plastic bag filled with flour and salt until chicken is coated.

Place chicken in a single layer in a shallow baking pan and bake for 25–30 minutes until cooked through.

While chicken is baking, combine oregano, thyme, basil, salt, paprika, and peppers, and set aside.

In a large frying pan, sauté garlic, onion, celery, green pepper, and tomato in oil. Add a splash of water and cook vegetables until soft.

Mix in seasoning mixture and let simmer for about a minute.

Mix in broth and tomato sauce. Bring to a boil, then simmer for 5 minutes.

Lower heat and add chicken breast, potato, and bay leaves. Cook until potatoes are tender.

NOTE: If you find the finished dish too "hot" for your taste, dilute with an additional can of tomato sauce.

*8 servings*
*Calories per serving: 196 total; 28 fat; 2 sat-fat*

# CHINESE CHICKEN

¼ cup + 2 tablespoons soy sauce (approximately)

¼ cup dry sherry

1 clove garlic

3 or 4 shakes ground ginger or 1 thin slice ginger root

½ cup + 1 tablespoon sugar (approximately)

5–6 star anise*

2 cups water (approximately)

10 boneless, skinless chicken breasts**

2 tablespoons soy sauce

1 tablespoon sugar

Place ¼ cup soy sauce, sherry, garlic, ginger, ½ cup sugar, star anise, and 1 cup of the water in an electric frying pan (or large frying pan). Add chicken in one layer and cook over medium heat for 20 minutes. Sauce will be thick.

Turn chicken. Add remaining 1 cup water, 2 tablespoons soy sauce, and 1 tablespoon sugar.

Taste. If too salty, add more sugar. If too sweet, add more soy sauce.

Cook for 10–30 minutes more or until chicken is cooked through. Keep adding water when sauce gets too thick. Periodically turn chicken. Keep tasting sauce and add soy sauce or sugar if necessary.

Chicken should be a deep brown.

*10 servings*

| Calories per serving: | Total | Fat | Sat-fat |
|---|---|---|---|
| 1 breast | 183 | 13 | 3 |
| 1 drumstick | 130 | 19 | 5 |
| 1 thigh | 134 | 24 | 5 |

---

*Available at Asian food stores and some supermarkets.

**You may substitute skinless chicken thighs or drumsticks for some of the chicken breasts.

# COQ AU VIN

2 whole frying chickens
¾ cup unbleached white flour
¼ teaspoon freshly ground black
　　pepper
¼ cup cognac or brandy
2 cups full-bodied red wine (*not*
　　hearty burgundy)
1 can (10¾ oz) chicken broth,
　　defatted
2 cloves garlic, minced

1 teaspoon salt (optional)
1 bay leaf
½ teaspoon thyme
12 small white onions, peeled
½–1 pound mushrooms
1 teaspoon olive oil
2 tablespoons margarine
3 tablespoons unbleached white
　　flour

Preheat oven to 375°F.

Cut chickens into parts and remove skin. If you cannot remove the skin from a part (such as the wings) do not use that part.

Put flour and pepper in a plastic bag. Add chicken and shake until coated. Place chicken in one layer in a shallow pan and bake until fully cooked, 20–30 minutes. Transfer to a large casserole.

Pour cognac over chicken and ignite it. Shake pan while cognac is burning. When flame subsides, add wine, chicken broth, garlic, salt, bay leaf, thyme, and onions and simmer, covered, until chicken is tender (about 25 minutes).

Remove chicken from casserole and cover to keep warm.

Boil liquid in casserole until it is reduced to about 3 cups (about 10 minutes). Remove from heat.

Sauté mushrooms in olive oil. Add a splash of water and cook mushrooms for about 1 minute and set aside.

Make a paste of the margarine and flour and mix into reduced liquid in casserole. Reheat slowly until liquid is thickened.

Return chicken and mushrooms to casserole and heat through.

Serve over noodles (shells, rotini, etc.).

*10 servings*

| Calories per serving: | Total | Fat | Sat-fat |
|---|---|---|---|
| 1 chicken breast | 195 | 35 | 9 |
| 1 drumstick | 140 | 41 | 10 |
| 1 thigh | 148 | 46 | 11 |

# CHICKEN COUSCOUS

3 boneless, skinless chicken
   breasts, cut into bite-size
   pieces
½ cup sliced carrot
¼ cup sliced celery
1 small turnip, quartered
½ cup dry white wine or
   vermouth
½ teaspoon thyme
¼ teaspoon rosemary
¼ teaspoon salt (optional)

¼ teaspoon paprika
1 tablespoon slivered almonds
1 cup sliced onion
2 teaspoons olive oil
½ teaspoon coriander
2 tablespoons raisins
¾ cup chopped tomatoes
½ teaspoon cinnamon
1 cup quick-cooking couscous
1 teaspoon margarine

In a large casserole, combine chicken, carrot, celery, turnip, wine, thyme, rosemary, salt, and paprika, with water to cover.

Bring to a boil, reduce heat, and simmer, covered, until chicken is cooked (about 10–20 minutes).

Meanwhile, in a medium skillet, toast almonds over low heat until golden. Remove almonds and set aside.

In same skillet, cook onion in olive oil over low heat, covered, until soft, stirring often.

Mix in coriander and raisins and cook slowly for 5 minutes more. Set aside.

When chicken is finished cooking, pour off and reserve all but about ½ cup of the liquid.

Add tomatoes and cinnamon to the chicken mixture and mix well. Cook, covered, for 5 minutes more.

Make couscous according to package directions. It takes about 5 minutes. (Add 1 teaspoon margarine instead of any amount of butter they suggest.)

Reheat onion-raisin mixture and sprinkle almonds over it.

Place couscous on a large platter. Cover with onions. Top with chicken and vegetables. Spoon on remaining sauce from casserole.

*5 servings*
*Calories per serving: 283 total; 24 fat; 9 sat-fat*

## CHICKEN WITH DRIED FRUIT AND LEMON

4 boneless, skinless chicken
   breasts
¼ cup chopped onion
1 tablespoon brown sugar
½ teaspoon ground ginger
¼–½ teaspoon salt (optional)
10 pitted prunes

2 tablespoons raisins
1 lemon, thinly sliced
¼ cup canned beef broth
¼ cup water
1 tablespoon soy sauce
1 tablespoon cornstarch

If you have a clay cooker, soak it in water for 15 minutes. Preheat oven to 450°F.

Place chicken in clay cooker or shallow baking pan.

Distribute onion evenly over chicken.

Combine sugar, ginger, and salt and spread half of the mixture over chicken.

Distribute prunes and raisins evenly over chicken.

Cover with lemon slices.

Sprinkle remaining sugar mixture over lemon.

Combine beef broth, water, and soy sauce and pour over chicken.

Cover clay cooker with top or cover baking pan tightly with aluminum foil.

Cook for 30–45 minutes or until chicken is cooked through.

Remove chicken to plate and cover with foil to keep warm.

Pour remaining liquid and fruit into small saucepan.

Mix cornstarch with about 2 tablespoons of liquid until smooth and add to saucepan. Heat until sauce thickens.

Serve chicken with fruited sauce.

*4 servings*
*Calories per serving: 226 total; 13 fat; 4 sat-fat*

# CHICKEN FAJITAS

4 boneless, skinless chicken breasts

### Marinade

2 cloves garlic, minced

1½ teaspoons cumin

½ teaspoon salt (optional)

3 tablespoons fresh lime juice

### Tomato Salsa

1 pound tomatoes, chopped

1 small onion, minced

1 fresh chili pepper, sliced thin

1 tablespoon fresh lime juice

### Vegetable Mélange

1 large onion, sliced

1 clove garlic, minced

1 green pepper, sliced

1 red or yellow sweet pepper, sliced

1 tablespoon olive oil

6 large flour tortillas*

Place chicken breasts in a bowl. Combine marinade ingredients and pour over chicken. Marinate in refrigerator at least 30 minutes.

Combine tomato salsa ingredients and refrigerate until ready to use.

Sauté onion, garlic, and peppers in olive oil until soft. Set aside.

Grill** or broil chicken breasts until cooked through. Slice into strips.

Warm the tortillas as directed on the package. They should be soft. (Don't bake them too long or you will have 6 very large crackers.)

To assemble each tortilla, lay pepper mixture across half, cover with chicken, and top with tomato salsa. Fold over top and serve.

*6 tortillas*
*Calories per serving: 212 total; 38 fat; 6 sat-fat*

---

*You may find tortillas in your grocery store in a refrigerated case. Look for tortillas with the least amount of fat. Do not use tortillas made with lard.
**Cast-iron griddles make great indoor grills.

# CHICKEN WITH FERMENTED BLACK BEANS AND NOODLES

3 ounces vermicelli rice noodles
About 1¼ pounds boneless,
    skinless chicken breasts
2 tablespoons fermented black
    beans*
1 tablespoon soy sauce
1 tablespoon vermouth
1 tablespoon vinegar
½ teaspoon five-spice powder
    (optional)

1 tablespoon ginger root
2 cloves garlic
1 green bell pepper
6 green onions
1 teaspoon olive oil
¼ cup water
1 can (14 oz) or bottle baby
    corns

Place noodles in a bowl and cover with water. Set aside.

Cut chicken into bite-size pieces and place in glass or ceramic container.

Combine soy sauce, vermouth, and 1 tablespoon of the fermented black beans and pour over chicken. Cover and refrigerate for about 20 minutes.

Combine remaining black beans, vinegar, and five-spice powder and set aside.

Mince ginger and garlic. Roughly cut green pepper into bite-size pieces. Slice green onions in half lengthwise, then cut into 1-inch pieces. Set aside.

In a wok or large skillet, sauté ginger and garlic in oil until fragrant.

Add chicken and marinade and cook, stirring constantly. Add water. When chicken is cooked through, add green peppers, green onions, and corn. Stir until vegetables are covered with sauce.

Mix in black-bean/vinegar mixture.

Drain noodles and stir in. Add more water if dish is too dry.

Serve over rice.

*6 servings*
*Calories per serving: 176 total; 26 fat; 5 sat-fat*

---

*Available at Asian food stores and some supermarkets.

# FIFTIES CHICKEN

¼ cup unbleached white flour
1 clove garlic, crushed
4 boneless, skinless chicken
  breasts
½ cup chopped onion
½ cup chopped green pepper

2 teaspoons olive oil
¾ cup orange juice
½ cup chili sauce
1 tablespoon Dijon mustard
1 tablespoon soy sauce

Preheat oven to 350°F.

Combine flour and garlic and place on a plate. Roll chicken pieces in flour, covering both sides. Place in shallow baking pan just large enough to hold pieces in one layer. Set aside.

Sauté onion and green pepper in olive oil until tender. Mix in orange juice, chili sauce, Dijon mustard, and soy sauce. Use half the sauce to cover chicken. Reserve the other half in refrigerator.

Bake chicken for 30–45 minutes or until cooked through. Heat reserved sauce and spoon over chicken.

*4 servings*
*Calories per serving: 200 total; 33 fat; 7 sat-fat*

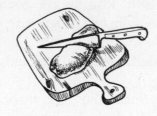

# GARLIC-BALSAMIC CHICKEN

One, two, three and you have a tasty, elegant entrée.

| | |
|---|---|
| 6 cloves garlic | ½ teaspoon freshly ground black |
| 1 can (10½ oz) chicken broth, | pepper |
|    defatted | ¼ teaspoon sage |
| ¼ teaspoon rosemary leaves | ¼ teaspoon ground ginger |
| 4 boneless, skinless chicken | 1 teaspoon olive oil |
|    breasts | ¼ teaspoon balsamic vinegar |

Mince 3 cloves garlic and combine with chicken broth and rosemary in a small saucepan.

Bring to a boil and simmer until broth is reduced by half — about ¾ cup.

Meanwhile, pound chicken breasts until about ½ inch thick. Set aside.

Mince remaining garlic. In a small bowl combine it with black pepper, sage, and ginger.

Rub both sides of chicken with garlic-spice mixture. Set aside.

Place oil in large skillet on high heat. Cook chicken for about 5 minutes on each side or until cooked through. Remove chicken and keep warm.

Pour chicken broth mixture into skillet. Add vinegar and heat until hot.

Spoon sauce over chicken.

*4 servings*
*Calories per serving: 150 total; 23 fat; 5 sat-fat*

## GINGER CHICKEN WITH GREEN ONIONS

5 boneless, skinless chicken
   breasts
1 teaspoon ground ginger
2 tablespoons cornstarch
1¼ cups water
3 tablespoons soy sauce
2 tablespoons olive oil

2 cloves garlic, minced
2 teaspoons minced ginger root
2 dried red peppers, crushed, or
   1 teaspoon dried red pepper
   flakes
1½ cups green onions cut into
   1-inch pieces

Cut chicken into bite-size pieces, sprinkle with ground ginger, and set aside for 15 minutes.

Make a smooth paste of the cornstarch and 2 tablespoons of the water. Stir in 2 more tablespoons of water and soy sauce. Set aside.

Sauté chicken in oil until cooked through.

Stir in garlic, ginger root, and red pepper flakes.

Mix in soy sauce mixture and heat until the sauce thickens.

If sauce is too thick, add remaining water, ¼ cup at a time, until desired consistency is achieved.

Stir in green onions and serve over rice.

*6 servings*
*Calories per serving: 172 total; 51 fat; 9 sat-fat*

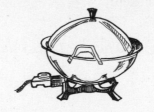

# HUNAN CHICKEN WITH ONIONS AND PEPPERS

4 boneless, skinless chicken
  breasts
½ cup unbleached white flour
½ teaspoon salt (optional)
¼ teaspoon freshly ground black
  pepper
2 tablespoons cornstarch
2 tablespoons + 1 cup water
3 tablespoons soy sauce
1 tablespoon dry sherry
3 tablespoons white vinegar

1 can (8 oz) water chestnuts
1 tablespoon olive oil
1 clove garlic, minced
2 medium onions, sliced (about
  1½ cups)
1 red pepper and 1 green pepper
  (or 2 green peppers), seeded
  and cut into strips
2–3 whole dried chili peppers,
  crumbled*

Preheat oven to 375°F.

Shake chicken in a plastic bag with flour, salt, and pepper until coated. Place chicken in a single layer in a baking pan and bake until fully cooked, about 20–30 minutes. When chicken is cool enough to handle, cut into bite-size pieces. Set aside.

Combine cornstarch with two tablespoons water. Stir in remaining cup of water. Set aside.

Combine soy sauce, sherry, and vinegar and set aside.

Heat olive oil in large skillet or wok. Sauté garlic, onions, red and green peppers, and water chestnuts on high heat for 1 minute, adding a splash of water as they begin to cook. Lower to medium and cook until soft but not limp. Add chili peppers.

Mix chicken into vegetables. Add sauce. Stir until chicken is well coated. Add cornstarch mixture. Stir until sauce thickens. If sauce is too thick, add water, a tablespoon at a time, until it reaches the right consistency.

Serve over rice.

*6 servings*
*Calories per serving: 162 total; 29 fat; 5 sat-fat*

*Do not crumble with bare fingers or you may burn your skin.

## INDONESIAN CHICKEN WITH GREEN BEANS

A beautiful dish — green beans set against ocher-colored sauce — and very tasty. You can substitute Chinese snow peas and ½ pound of sliced mushrooms for the beans and add them with the chicken as the last step.

6 boneless, skinless chicken
  breasts
½ cup unbleached white flour
¼ teaspoon black pepper
½ teaspoon salt (optional)
1 pound green beans, washed
  and cut into bite-size pieces
10 cloves garlic, minced
1 tablespoon minced ginger root

1 small onion, chopped
1 teaspoon olive oil
Juice of 1 lime
1 tablespoon double black soy
  sauce*
2 teaspoons brown sugar
2 teaspoons turmeric
1 teaspoon salt (optional)
½ cup water

Preheat oven to 375°F.

Shake chicken in a plastic bag with flour, pepper, and salt.

Place chicken in a single layer in a baking pan and bake until fully cooked, about 20–30 minutes. Set aside. You may bake the chicken the night before and refrigerate it until ready to add to sauce.

Cook green beans in a pot of boiling water for 5–10 minutes until tender but still crisp. Set aside.

Cut chicken into bite-size pieces. Set aside.

Sauté garlic, ginger, and onion in olive oil until soft.

Add lime juice, soy sauce, brown sugar, turmeric, and ¼ cup of the water.

Slowly add remaining water, if sauce is too thick.

Add chicken and green beans and stir until completely covered with sauce.

Serve over rice.

*8 servings*
*Calories per serving: 135 total; 14 fat; 4 sat-fat*

---

*Double black soy sauce is available at Asian food stores and some supermarkets. You can make your own by mixing 2 teaspoons soy sauce with 1 teaspoon dark molasses.

# INDONESIAN PEANUT CHICKEN

Peanuts are a major ingredient in Indonesian cooking. The spicy peanut sauce that covers this chicken dish is called a satay.

4 boneless, skinless chicken
  breasts
½ cup unbleached white flour

½ teaspoon salt (optional)
¼ teaspoon freshly ground black
  pepper

*Satay sauce*

1 clove garlic
1 small onion
1 teaspoon ginger root
⅓ cup shelled roasted peanuts,
  unsalted
2 teaspoons soy sauce
2 teaspoons turmeric

1½ teaspoons lime (preferred) or
  lemon juice
1–2 hot chili peppers
¾ cup water
1 large onion, sliced
1 teaspoon olive oil

Preheat oven to 375°F.

Shake chicken in a plastic bag with flour, salt, and pepper.

Place chicken in a single layer in a shallow baking pan and bake until fully cooked, 20–30 minutes. Set aside and make satay. You may bake the chicken the night before and refrigerate it until ready to use.

Blend garlic, onion, ginger, peanuts, soy sauce, turmeric, lime or lemon juice, chili peppers, and water in blender or food processor until smooth.

Place sauce in top of double boiler and heat water to boiling. Cover pot and cook sauce for 10–20 minutes or until thick.

Sauté onion rings in olive oil until soft.

Cut chicken into bite-size pieces and warm in a large skillet.

Pour satay sauce over chicken and stir until chicken is well coated. If sauce is too thick, add a small amount of water, 1 tablespoon at a time.

Stir in onion rings and serve over rice.

*5 servings*
*Calories per serving: 148 total; 61 fat; 10 sat-fat*

# JAMBALAYA

This delicious, colorful dish may be used as a main course. Or you can eliminate the chicken and shrimp and serve it as a side dish. Eat it hot the first day and cool the next.

½ pound shrimp
1 boneless, skinless chicken
    breast
2 stalks celery, diced
1 medium green pepper, diced
1 teaspoon olive oil
1½ cups long-grain rice
¼ teaspoon salt (optional)
½ teaspoon oregano

¼ teaspoon cayenne pepper
¼ teaspoon freshly ground black
    pepper
1 bay leaf
1 can (10¾ oz) chicken broth,
    defatted
2¼ cups water
1–2 large red peppers, diced

Shell and devein shrimp. Set aside.

Cut chicken breast into bite-size pieces. Set aside.

In a large casserole or saucepan, sauté celery and green peppers in olive oil.

Add rice, salt, oregano, cayenne, black pepper, and bay leaf and stir for a few seconds.

Pour in chicken broth and water. Bring to a boil.

Add shrimp, chicken, and red peppers. Cover, turn heat to low, and cook for about 20 minutes or until rice is tender. All of the liquid should *not* be absorbed; if it is, the dish will be too dry.

*7 one-cup servings*
*Calories per serving: 221 total; 13 fat; 3 sat-fat*

# KEEMA MATAR

Traditionally, Keema Matar is made with ground lamb or beef. It tastes equally good with ground chicken, and instead of spending 254 fat calories on ground lean beef, you spend a mere 14. Serve Keema Matar over Indian Rice (page 193) for a superb combination of flavors.

1½ pounds boneless, skinless
  chicken breasts
1 tablespoon olive oil
1 tablespoon water
1 tablespoon minced garlic
  (about 4–5 cloves)

2–3 tablespoons curry powder
1 cinnamon stick
½ teaspoon salt (optional)
1 cup frozen peas
1–2 tablespoons water

If you are planning to make Indian Rice, prepare it first.

Grind chicken breasts in a food processor or a meat grinder. If you are using a food processor, first cut the cold (but not frozen) chicken breasts into 1-inch cubes. Place cubes in the work bowl. Press the Pulse/Off button until chicken is ground (not puréed!).

In a large skillet or wok, sauté chicken in olive oil, stirring constantly. Add water. Continue stirring until chicken is cooked through.

Mix in garlic, curry powder, cinnamon stick, and salt.

Add peas and stir until heated through. Mix in water if chicken is too dry.

Serve over Indian Rice.

*5 servings*
*Calories per serving: 200 total; 38 fat; 8 sat-fat*

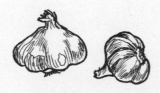

# CHICKEN KIEV

This recipe is a gem: it uses ingredients you probably have on hand; it takes no time to make; and the resulting dish is so special you can proudly serve it to the most discriminating of guests.

| | |
|---|---|
| 1 clove garlic, finely chopped | 4 boneless, skinless chicken |
| ½ teaspoon basil |    breasts |
| ½ teaspoon oregano | 1 tablespoon margarine |
| ¼ teaspoon salt (optional) | 3 tablespoons dry white wine or |
| 1 cup fine bread crumbs made |    vermouth |
|    from 1–2 slices of white bread | ¼ cup sliced green onions |
|    or challah* | |

Preheat oven to 375°F.

Mix garlic, basil, oregano, and salt with bread crumbs and place on a large plate. (You can mince the garlic in a food processor, add bread and process until it becomes crumbs, then add spices and process again.)

Roll each chicken breast in bread crumbs and place it in a shallow baking pan.

Bake near center of oven for 30–45 minutes or until fully cooked.

Melt the margarine. Mix in wine and green onions.

Pour sauce over chicken.

Return chicken to oven for 3–5 minutes or until sauce is hot. Serve over rice.

*4 servings*
*Calories per serving: 175 total; 38 fat; 6 sat-fat*

---

*Avoid commercial bread crumbs. It is less expensive and healthier to make your own crumbs from a few slices of bread.

# KUNG PAO CHICKEN WITH BROCCOLI

You can easily make Chinese cooking low-fat by limiting the amount of oil you use or by flouring and baking the chicken first and adding it to the sauce. It still tastes delicious.

4 boneless, skinless chicken
  breasts
¼ cup unbleached white flour
¼ teaspoon salt (optional)
2 tablespoons cornstarch
2 tablespoons + 1 cup water
2 tablespoons bean sauce*
1 tablespoon hoison sauce*
1–2 teaspoons chili paste with
  garlic*

½ teaspoon sugar
1 tablespoon sherry
1 tablespoon white vinegar
2 cloves garlic, peeled and
  flattened
1 head broccoli, stem trimmed,
  cut into flowerets
2 tablespoons unsalted roasted
  peanuts, shelled
1–3 dried hot red peppers

Preheat oven to 375°F.

Shake chicken in a plastic bag with flour and salt until coated. Place chicken in a single layer in a baking pan and bake until fully cooked, about 20–30 minutes. When chicken is cool enough to handle, cut it into bite-size pieces. Set aside.

Meanwhile, combine cornstarch with 2 tablespoons water. Stir in remaining cup of water. Set aside.

Combine bean sauce, hoisin sauce, chili paste with garlic, sugar, sherry, vinegar, and garlic and set aside.

Steam broccoli in wok or saucepan until tender. Set aside.

Heat chicken in wok or large skillet. Add sauce. Stir until chicken is well coated. Add cornstarch mixture.

When sauce thickens, stir in peanuts and red peppers. Add broccoli and mix until well coated with sauce.

Mix in ¼–½ cup water if sauce is too dry.

Serve over rice.

*6 servings*
*Calories per serving: 140 total; 24 fat; 2 sat-fat*

*Available at Asian food stores and some supermarkets.

# LEMON CHICKEN

A delicate blending of tart and sweet, Lemon Chicken can't help but become one of your most popular family or company dishes.

4 boneless, skinless chicken
  breasts
Juice of 1 lemon
¼ cup unbleached white flour
¼ teaspoon freshly ground black
  pepper
½ teaspoon salt (optional)

¼ teaspoon paprika
1½ tablespoons grated lemon
  peel
3 tablespoons brown sugar
3 tablespoons lemon juice
1 tablespoon water
1 lemon, sliced thin

Place chicken in a bowl or casserole. Pour lemon juice over breasts and marinate in refrigerator for several hours or overnight, turning chicken periodically.

Preheat oven to 350°F.

Combine flour, pepper, salt, and paprika in plastic bag.

Remove chicken breasts from marinade and coat each with flour by shaking it in the plastic bag.

Place chicken in a baking pan in a single layer.

Either peel the yellow (zest) from a lemon and chop it fine in your food processor (a mini food chopper makes a perfect grater), or grate the zest with a hand grater. Mix 1 tablespoon of the grated peel with the brown sugar.

Sprinkle the lemon zest–sugar mixture evenly over the chicken breasts. Combine 3 tablespoons lemon juice and water and sprinkle evenly over chicken.

Put 1 lemon slice on each chicken breast and bake chicken for 35–40 minutes or until cooked through.

*4 servings*
*Calories per serving: 176 total; 13 fat; 4 sat-fat*

## LEMON-MUSTARD CHICKEN

4 boneless, skinless chicken
   breasts
2 teaspoons margarine
1½ tablespoons Dijon mustard

2 tablespoons fresh lemon juice
½ teaspoon tarragon
¼ teaspoon salt (optional)

Preheat oven to 375°F.

Place chicken in a shallow baking pan.

In a small saucepan, melt margarine. Stir in mustard, lemon juice, tarragon, and salt. Pour over chicken.

Bake chicken for 30–45 minutes or until cooked through.

Spoon sauce from pan over chicken.

*4 servings*
*Calories per serving: 147 total; 28 fat; 6 sat-fat*

## CHICKEN MARRAKESH

4 boneless, skinless chicken
   breasts
3 tablespoons fresh lemon juice
1 tablespoon grated lemon peel
1 clove garlic, minced

2–3 teaspoons thyme
½ teaspoon salt (optional)
½ teaspoon freshly ground black
   pepper
1 lemon, thinly sliced

Place chicken in a bowl or casserole.

Mix together lemon juice, lemon peel, garlic, thyme, salt, and pepper and pour over chicken. Marinate chicken in refrigerator for at least 3 hours.

Preheat oven to 350°F.

Remove chicken from marinade and place in shallow baking dish.

Pour marinade over chicken and bake chicken for 30–45 minutes or until cooked through.

Garnish with lemon slices.

*4 servings*
*Calories per serving: 132 total; 13 fat; 4 sat-fat*

## LIME-PEANUT-GINGER CHICKEN

Don't be put off by our ho-hum name for this chicken recipe. Although it contains these three ingredients (actually peanut butter), the flavors combine to produce a unique and simply delectable taste.

6 boneless, skinless chicken
   breasts
½ cup fresh lime juice
1 clove garlic
1 tablespoon sliced ginger root
1 teaspoon whole black
   peppercorns
1 teaspoon dried basil
1 tablespoon soy sauce
1 tablespoon white vinegar
1 teaspoon honey

1 tablespoon water
1 tablespoon grated lemon peel
2 tablespoons olive oil
1 tablespoon sesame oil
1 tablespoon natural all-peanut
   peanut butter
2–3 cups sliced mushrooms
1 tablespoon cornstarch diluted
   in 2 tablespoons water
¼–½ cup sliced green onions

Cut chicken into bite-size pieces and marinate in lime juice for at least 2 hours in refrigerator.

Make a dressing by chopping garlic, ginger, and peppercorns in food processor or blender until pepper is no longer whole. (It will probably be impossible to break up all the peppercorns.)

Blend in basil, soy sauce, vinegar, honey, water, and grated lemon peel.

Pour 1 tablespoon of the olive oil into the processor or blender and process until smooth. Set dressing aside.

Remove chicken from marinade and sauté it in sesame oil and the remaining tablespoon of olive oil until it turns white.

Add dressing and stir until chicken is well coated and sauce is warm.

Mix in peanut butter. Stir in mushrooms. Add cornstarch mixture to thicken sauce.

Sprinkle green onions on top and serve over rice.

*8 servings*
*Calories per serving: 175 total; 64 fat; 11 sat-fat*

# MA-PO BEAN CURD

This is not a beautiful dish, but it is extremely tasty and easy.

1 teaspoon olive oil

1 tablespoon minced ginger root

2 boneless, skinless chicken breasts, ground (can be ground in food processor)

2 tablespoons water

16 ounces tofu (fresh bean curd),* cubed

½ cup water

1½–3 tablespoons soy sauce

½ teaspoon sugar

1–3 teaspoons chili paste with garlic*

1 tablespoon fermented black beans*

1 tablespoon cornstarch mixed with 2 tablespoons water

½ tablespoon sesame oil*

2 tablespoons sliced green onion

Heat a wok or large skillet until hot. Add olive oil and sauté ginger until fragrant (about 10 seconds).

Add chicken and stir until it turns white. Add water to help cook chicken.

Stir in tofu, water, 1½ tablespoons of the soy sauce, and sugar.

Reduce heat, cover, and simmer for 5–10 minutes.

Uncover and stir in chili paste with garlic and fermented black beans.

Raise heat and stir in cornstarch mixture and sesame oil until sauce thickens. Taste. Add remaining soy sauce, a teaspoon at a time, if needed for flavor.

Stir in green onion and serve over rice.

*6 servings*
*Calories per serving: 130 total; 53 fat; 8 sat-fat*

*Available at Asian food stores and some supermarkets.

# MONGOLIAN HOT POT

Making this dish is a group activity that allows each person to be a cook. It works like a fondue. Everyone skewers a piece of meat or vegetable and dips it into simmering broth in a large Oriental "hot pot" or in an electric frying pan or wok. When the meat is finished cooking, the enriched broth becomes an after-dinner soup.

6 boneless, skinless chicken breasts

### Marinade

| | |
|---|---|
| 2 cloves garlic, minced | 2 tablespoons honey |
| 1 teaspoon olive oil | ¼ cup soy sauce |
| 1 tablespoon white vinegar | 1 teaspoon sherry |

### Sauce

| | |
|---|---|
| ½ cup soy sauce | 2 tablespoons minced ginger |
| ½ cup dry sherry | root |
| 5 tablespoons honey | 2 cloves garlic, minced |

### The Rest

| | |
|---|---|
| 4 ounces cellophane noodles* | ½ head celery cabbage, coarsely |
| ½ pound snow peas | chopped |
| 1 zucchini, cut into ¼-inch slices | 1 pound bay scallops |

### Broth

| | |
|---|---|
| 10 cups chicken stock, or 2 cans | 3 green onions, sliced |
| (10¾ oz each) chicken broth, | 1½ teaspoons sliced ginger root |
| defatted, + 6 cans water | 2 cloves garlic, minced |

4 cups hot cooked rice

Slice chicken breasts into slender, bite-size pieces. Marinate in garlic, olive oil, vinegar, honey, soy sauce, and sherry in refrigerator for several hours or overnight.

---

*Available at Asian food stores and some supermarkets.

Mix all sauce ingredients together and set aside.

Pour boiling water over cellophane noodles and let stand for 5–10 minutes or until soft. Drain and set aside.

Remove chicken from marinade and arrange artistically on a plate.

Arrange another plate with snow peas, zucchini slices, and celery cabbage. Set aside.

Arrange bay scallops on another plate.

Pour chicken broth and water into a hot pot, chafing dish, or electric wok or frying pan set in the center of the table. Heat to a slow boil.

Mix in green onions, ginger, and garlic.

Give each person a bowl of rice, a plate, and a small custard dish for the sauce. Pass around the trays of chicken, scallops, and vegetables so people may take what they wish. Each person should also have a fondue fork, skewer, or sharp implement to dip chicken, scallops, and vegetables in broth until cooked.

When food has been devoured or everyone is almost full, add noodles and celery cabbage to the broth and cook for 2–3 minutes.

Serve resulting soup in bowls.

*8 servings*

| *Calories per serving:* | *Total* | *Fat* | *Sat-fat* |
|---|---|---|---|
| 2 tablespoons sauce | 69 | 0 | 0 |
| Meat and vegetables | 155 | 25 | 4 |
| Broth | 184 | 0 | 0 |
| Total | 408 | 25 | 4 |

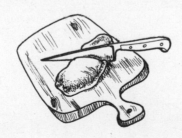

## GRAINY MUSTARD CHICKEN

This simple, elegant dish could not be simpler to make. The recipe is for 4 breasts, but you could just as easily make 20. Just increase the mustard, honey, and soy sauce in the same proportions to accommodate larger amounts.

4 boneless, skinless chicken
   breasts
3 tablespoons grainy Dijon
   mustard*

3 tablespoons honey
1½ teaspoons soy sauce

Place chicken breasts in a glass or ceramic container.

In a small bowl, mix mustard, honey, and soy sauce.

Spoon 3 tablespoons of the mustard mixture over chicken, making sure all surfaces are covered, and refrigerate the rest to use later. Marinate for at least 20 minutes but preferably for several hours in the refrigerator.

Preheat the broiler for about 10 minutes.

Place breasts in one layer on a broiler pan. Pour remaining marinade and reserved sauce over them.

Broil about 3–4 inches from the heating coil for 10–15 minutes, checking to see if done after 10 minutes.

*4 servings*
*Calories per serving: 193 total; 19 fat; 4 sat-fat*

---

*We use Maille L'Ancienne Dijon Mustard. Choose a Dijon mustard that is full of seeds.

## CHICKEN NUGGETS CHEZ GOOR

The chicken nuggets that you get at fast-food chains are deep-fried in highly saturated oils. Instead of devouring 200 fat calories (8 Mc-Nuggets), make Chicken Nuggets Chez Goor (43 fat calories).

4 boneless, skinless chicken
  breasts
1 tablespoon olive oil
2 cloves garlic, minced
¼ teaspoon freshly ground black
  pepper

1 cup finely ground bread
  crumbs, made from 2–3 slices
  French or other bread
¼ teaspoon cayenne pepper
2½ teaspoons honey
2 tablespoons Dijon mustard

Preheat oven to 375°F.

Cut each chicken breast into 8 pieces.

Mix oil, garlic, and pepper with chicken pieces and marinate about 30 minutes.

Combine bread crumbs and cayenne and place on plate.

Roll chicken pieces in bread crumbs and place on large cookie sheet in a single layer.

Bake for about 15 minutes until browned and cooked through. For extra browning, broil for a few more minutes.

Combine honey and mustard. Dip nuggets into honey-mustard sauce.

*4 servings*

| Calories per serving: | Total | Fat | Sat-fat |
|---|---|---|---|
| | 191 | 43 | 5 |
| With honey-mustard sauce | 211 | 43 | 5 |

## CHINESE CHICKEN WITH ORANGES

4 boneless, skinless chicken
   breasts
2 tablespoons soy sauce
1½ tablespoons cornstarch
½ tablespoon hoisin sauce*
3 tablespoons dry sherry
1 cup water
1 clove garlic, minced

1 teaspoon minced ginger root
2 tablespoons orange peel slivers
½ teaspoon olive oil
1 teaspoon marmalade
½–1 teaspoon red pepper flakes
1 orange, peeled and cut into
   bite-size pieces
10–20 snow peas

Place chicken between two pieces of wax paper and pound with a meat mallet to flatten. Then steam in a vegetable steamer or on a steamer tray in a wok until cooked through. Pull or slice chicken into thin strips about 2–3 inches long.

Mix soy sauce into cornstarch, a tablespoon at a time, creating a smooth paste.

Mix in hoisin sauce, sherry, and water, and set aside.

Sauté garlic, ginger, and orange peel slivers in oil until soft.

Stir in cooked chicken pieces.

Stir in cornstarch mixture and cook until it thickens. Add more water if too dry.

Mix in marmalade, red pepper flakes, orange pieces, and snow peas and heat. Serve over rice.

*6 servings*
*Calories per serving: 119 total; 12 fat; 4 sat-fat*

---

*Available at Asian food stores and some supermarkets.

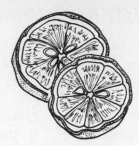

# ORANGE CHICKEN CHINOISE

6 boneless, skinless chicken
    breasts
1 tablespoon minced orange
    zest*
1½ tablespoons hoisin sauce**
2 teaspoons chili paste with
    garlic**

2 tablespoons soy sauce
2 tablespoons orange
    marmalade
2 cloves garlic, minced
½ cup orange juice
1 teaspoon cornstarch

Place chicken in a glass or ceramic container.

In a small bowl or jar, combine remaining ingredients except corn-starch. Spoon ¼ cup of marinade evenly over chicken breasts and re-frigerate the rest to use later. Cover container and marinate chicken several hours or overnight in the refrigerator.

Preheat broiler.

Take chicken breasts from marinade and place in a single row on a broiler pan. Broil chicken for 10 minutes or until cooked through.

Pour reserved marinade into small saucepan. Stir in cornstarch. Heat until thick.

Spoon sauce over chicken breasts.

*6 servings*
*Calories per serving: 177 total; 15 fat; 4 sat-fat*

---

*A convenient way to make minced orange zest is to use either a zester or a knife to re-move the orange part of the peel (not the white underneath), then place zest in mini-chopper and chop until fine. You may also use a grater.
**Available at Asian food stores or in the Asian foods aisle of the grocery store.

# CHICKEN PAPRIKASH

Paprikash dishes typically use sour cream. Nonfat yogurt is used here without affecting the taste. Half a cup of nonfat yogurt contains 0 fat calories. Half a cup of sour cream contains 217 fat calories.

| | |
|---|---|
| ½ cup unbleached white flour | 2 teaspoons olive oil |
| ½–1 teaspoon salt (optional) | 1½ teaspoons paprika |
| ¼ teaspoon freshly ground black pepper | ½ teaspoon dillweed |
| | ½ teaspoon salt |
| 6 boneless, skinless chicken breasts | ¼ teaspoon freshly ground black pepper |
| 3 tablespoons water | 1 cup chicken broth, defatted |
| 1½ tablespoons cornstarch | ½ cup nonfat yogurt |
| ½ cup chopped onion | ½–1 cup water |
| 2–3 cups sliced mushrooms | |

Preheat oven to 375°F.

Place flour, ½–1 teaspoon salt, and ¼ teaspoon pepper in a plastic bag. Piece by piece, coat chicken by shaking it in the bag.

Arrange floured chicken in one layer in a shallow baking pan and bake for 30–40 minutes or until chicken is cooked through.

In a small bowl, add water to cornstarch and mix until smooth. Set aside.

Meanwhile, in a large skillet, sauté onion and mushrooms in oil. Add a splash of water and cook vegetables until tender.

Stir in paprika, dillweed, ½ teaspoon salt, ¼ teaspoon pepper, and chicken broth.

Add cornstarch mixture and bring to a boil, stirring constantly. Lower heat to medium.

Cut chicken into bite-size pieces and add to sauce. Stir until chicken is heated.

Remove from heat and stir in yogurt. Add water, ¼ cup at a time, if sauce is too thick.

Serve over rice or noodles.

*8 servings*
*Calories per serving: 152 total; 23 fat; 5 sat-fat*

# PEPPERY CHICKEN

A very peppery chicken that tastes good grilled or roasted in the oven.

4 boneless, skinless chicken
  breasts
2 tablespoons soy sauce
2 tablespoons honey
½ teaspoon thyme
½ teaspoon paprika

¼ teaspoon cayenne pepper
1 tablespoon white vinegar
½ teaspoon allspice
1 teaspoon freshly ground black
  pepper
1 cup sliced mushrooms

Place chicken in a shallow casserole.

Combine soy sauce, honey, thyme, paprika, cayenne pepper, vinegar, allspice, and pepper and pour over chicken. Marinate in refrigerator for about 1 hour.

### To Bake

Preheat oven to 375°F.

Bake chicken for 30–45 minutes or until cooked through.

Surround chicken with sliced mushrooms, spoon the sauce over them, and bake 1 minute more.

### To Grill

Remove breasts from marinade and grill until cooked through, basting periodically with marinade.

Add mushrooms to the marinade and simmer for 1 minute. Spoon over grilled chicken breasts.

*4 servings*
*Calories per serving: 172 total; 13 fat; 4 sat-fat*

# PHYLLO-WRAPPED CHICKEN WITH RICE, ARTICHOKES, AND CREAM SAUCE

What a wonderful combination of tastes and textures! This very elegant chicken can be made a day ahead and refrigerated. (We recommend that you do make this dish ahead because it involves many steps. To cook it along with all the other dishes that comprise a dinner will make you a nervous wreck and frazzled host.)

Phyllo dough that has been stored in the freezer has to be thawed in the refrigerator for 8 hours or overnight and then set out at room temperature for 2–4 hours before using. Take this into account when planning to cook this dish.

### Chicken

10 boneless, skinless chicken breasts
1 cup dry white wine or vermouth

1 teaspoon salt (optional)
1½ teaspoons thyme
½ teaspoon rosemary
1 bay leaf

### Rice

1 tablespoon margarine
2 cloves garlic, minced
½ cup chopped onion

½ pound sliced mushrooms
¾ cup long-grain rice

### Cream Sauce

2 tablespoons margarine
¼ cup unbleached white flour

½ cup skim milk

### Assembly

1 package (9 oz) frozen artichoke hearts, thawed, or 1 jar (11½ oz) artichoke hearts, packed in water and drained

3 tablespoons margarine
16 sheets phyllo dough,* thawed (usually comes in 16-oz package)

*Available at Greek or Mideastern food stores or in the freezer section of many supermarkets.

### The Chicken and Broth

In a large pot, combine chicken, wine, salt, thyme, rosemary, bay leaf, and water to cover. Bring to a boil. Reduce heat, cover, and simmer for 25 minutes or until chicken is cooked through.

Remove chicken and cut into bite-size pieces. Set aside.

Boil chicken broth gently, uncovered, until it is reduced to about 3½ cups.

Set aside and make the rice.

### The Rice

In a large saucepan, melt margarine.

Add garlic, onion, and mushrooms and cook until tender.

Stir in rice.

Add 1½ cups of the reduced chicken broth. Simmer, covered, until liquid is absorbed (about 20 minutes).

While rice is cooking, make cream sauce.

### The Cream Sauce

Melt margarine over low heat.

Stir in flour and cook until bubbly.

Remove from heat and slowly stir in remaining 2 cups of broth.

Gradually add skim milk. Return to low heat and stir until thick.

### The Rice and Chicken

When rice is cooked, stir in artichoke hearts and 1 cup of the cream sauce. Set aside.

Stir remaining cream sauce into chicken pieces. Set aside.

### Putting It All Together

Preheat oven to 350°F.

Grease a 13×9-inch baking pan with margarine.

Melt the 3 tablespoons margarine.

Unfold phyllo leaves. Cover with plastic or damp towel.

Place 1 phyllo sheet on bottom of pan. Brush lightly with melted margarine.

Repeat procedure with 6 more sheets of phyllo.

Spread half of rice mixture over phyllo dough.

Spread chicken over rice mixture.

Spread remaining rice mixture over chicken.

Cover with 6 sheets of phyllo, brushing with margarine between each sheet.

Tuck in edges of last sheet and brush top with margarine.

Cut lightly through 3 or 4 layers of phyllo dough to indicate pieces to be cut later.

Bake chicken for 30–45 minutes or until golden brown and bubbly. Or refrigerate for up to 24 hours and bake later for 60 minutes.

*12 servings*
*Calories per serving: 270 total; 56 fat; 12 sat-fat*

# CREAMY CHICKEN PIE

This chicken pie is a rich and creamy splurge.

Fully baked nonsweet pie crust
 (page 276)
½ cup chopped onion
3 cups sliced mushrooms
2 teaspoons olive oil
3 tablespoons unbleached white
 flour
1 cup low-fat (1%) cottage
 cheese

2 cups diced cooked chicken or
 turkey breast
⅓ cup chopped parsley
¼ teaspoon freshly ground black
 pepper
¼ teaspoon rosemary

Preheat oven to 375°F.

In a large skillet, sauté onion and mushrooms in olive oil over medium heat until most liquid has evaporated.

Stir in flour. Remove skillet from heat.

Stir in cottage cheese, chicken, parsley, pepper, and rosemary.

Spoon chicken mixture into pie shell. Cover with foil and cook for 10 minutes.

Remove foil and bake for 15 minutes or until crust is golden brown.

*7 servings*
*Calories per serving: 156 total; 60 fat; 11 sat-fat*

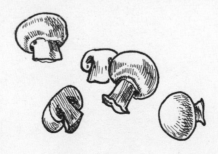

# PINEAPPLE CHICKEN

½ cup unbleached white flour
½ teaspoon salt (optional)
½ teaspoon paprika
¼ teaspoon freshly ground black
  pepper
4 boneless, skinless chicken
  breasts

1 cup pineapple chunks in heavy
  syrup*
½ cup heavy syrup
½ cup sliced green pepper
2 green onions, sliced
1½ teaspoons brown sugar
2 tablespoons dry sherry

Preheat oven to 425°F.

Combine flour, salt, paprika, and pepper in a plastic bag.

Piece by piece, coat chicken by shaking it in the bag.

Arrange floured chicken in a shallow baking pan in one layer. Bake at 425°F for 20 minutes. Turn chicken.

Combine pineapple, syrup, green pepper, green onions, brown sugar, and sherry and pour over chicken.

Lower heat to 375°F and bake until chicken is golden brown and sauce is thick (about 15–30 minutes).

*8 servings*
*Calories per serving: 210 total; 13 fat; 4 sat-fat*

---

*If possible, use pineapple in heavy syrup, not in its own juice. It may come only in a 20-ounce can. If so, drain the syrup from the can (reserve ½ cup) and set aside one cup of pineapple chunks.

# CHICKEN WITH RICE, TOMATOES, AND ARTICHOKES

3 boneless, skinless chicken
   breasts
2 cloves garlic, minced
½ cup chopped onion
1 teaspoon olive oil
1 large can (28 oz) tomatoes,
   chopped
2 cups water
½ teaspoon thyme

½ teaspoon oregano
1 teaspoon salt (optional)
¼ teaspoon freshly ground black
   pepper
1 bay leaf
1½ cups uncooked long-grain
   rice
1 jar (11½ oz) artichoke hearts,
   packed in water

Cut chicken into bite-size pieces and set aside.

In a large casserole, sauté garlic and onion in olive oil. Add a splash of water and cook vegetables until soft.

Stir in tomatoes and their liquid, water, thyme, oregano, salt, pepper, and bay leaf and bring to a boil.

Add chicken and rice, cover casserole, and reduce heat to low.

Cook for 25 minutes or until rice is tender, most liquid is absorbed, and chicken is cooked through.

Stir in artichokes and serve.

*8 one-cup servings*
*Calories per serving: 220 total; 15 fat; 3 sat-fat*

# SATE AJAM
## (Broiled Chicken on Skewers)

4 boneless, skinless chicken
 breasts
12 medium mushrooms
1 teaspoon olive oil
2 tablespoons fresh lime juice

⅛ teaspoon freshly ground black
 pepper
1 teaspoon cumin
1 teaspoon minced garlic

Cut chicken into 1-inch pieces and cut stems off mushrooms.

Alternate pieces of chicken with mushrooms on skewers. (Push skewers through the *tops* of the mushrooms to keep them from splitting.)

Place skewered chicken in a shallow casserole.

Combine olive oil, lime juice, pepper, cumin, and garlic and pour over chicken.

Turn skewers to coat chicken and mushrooms with oil mixture.

Refrigerate for at least 30 minutes.

Preheat broiler.

Place skewers on broiler pan and broil 6 inches from heat for about 10 minutes or until cooked through. Turn and baste several times.

Serve over rice and spoon warm marinade over chicken pieces.

*4 servings*
*Calories per serving: 151 total; 23 fat; 5 sat-fat*

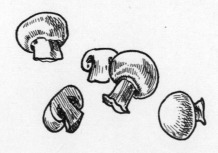

# SEOUL CHICKEN

3 tablespoons soy sauce
1 tablespoon + 1 teaspoon
    honey
1 tablespoon minced garlic
1 tablespoon minced fresh
    ginger
½–1 teaspoon freshly ground
    black pepper

¼ cup sliced green onions
1 teaspoon dark sesame oil (or 1
    teaspoon olive oil + ½
    teaspoon sesame seeds)
1½–2 cups carrots cut in 2-inch
    julienne strips*
4 boneless, skinless chicken
    breasts

Combine soy sauce, honey, garlic, ginger, and black pepper. Mix in green onions and set aside.

Heat oil in large skillet (or, if using sesame seeds and oil, combine and heat in large skillet until seeds begin to brown).

Add carrots and stir.

Stir in soy sauce mixture.

Place chicken breasts in skillet in one layer, turning each so it is completely covered with sauce.

Cover skillet and lower heat to medium.

Cook for 5 minutes, then turn chicken. Turn again in 5 minutes. If chicken is not finished cooking, turn again and cook until done.

*4 servings*
*Calories per serving: 192 total; 23 fat; 6 sat-fat*

---

*For directions on how to cut vegetable matchsticks, see page 166.

## SESAME CHICKEN BROCHETTES

6 boneless, skinless chicken
  breasts
¼ cup soy sauce
½ cup dry white wine or
  vermouth

1 clove garlic, minced
1 tablespoon sesame seeds,
  lightly toasted

Cut chicken breasts into 1-inch cubes and place in a bowl or casserole.

Combine soy sauce, wine, and garlic and pour over chicken. Marinate in refrigerator for at least 30 minutes.

Preheat oven to broil or prepare grill.

Remove chicken from marinade and reserve marinade.

Skewer chicken and broil or grill until cooked through, basting occasionally with marinade.

Sprinkle sesame seeds over chicken and serve over rice.

Heat marinade and spoon over chicken and rice.

*6 servings*
*Calories per serving: 160 total; 20 fat; 5 sat-fat*

# SHEPHERD'S CHICKEN CHILI PIE

1½–2 pounds potatoes, peeled
  and cut into chunks
4 boneless, skinless chicken
  breasts
1 can (16 oz) whole tomatoes,
  with juice
1 large onion, sliced
3 cloves garlic, minced
1 teaspoon olive oil

1½ tablespoons chili powder
½ teaspoon oregano
1 teaspoon cumin
2 tablespoons water
1 tablespoon tomato paste
1 teaspoon margarine
Salt and freshly ground black
  pepper to taste
1 tablespoon skim milk

Place potatoes in a saucepan with water to cover, bring to a boil, and simmer for about 10–15 minutes or until tender.

Steam chicken pieces in a vegetable steamer or on a steamer tray in a wok until cooked through, about 10 minutes.

Drain tomatoes. Reserve liquid.

Preheat oven to 350°F.

In a large skillet, sauté onion and garlic in olive oil until soft.

Mix in chili powder, oregano, and cumin.

Add water, tomato paste, and tomatoes. Cook until sauce is thick. If sauce becomes *too* thick, add a few tablespoons of the reserved tomato juice.

Mix chicken cubes into sauce.

Drain potatoes and whip them. Add margarine, salt, and pepper. Add skim milk and mix until potatoes are smooth. Add more milk if necessary.

Place chicken mixture in a shallow casserole. Spread potatoes on top. Bake for about 30 minutes.

*6 servings*
*Calories per serving: 204 total; 15 fat; 4 sat-fat*

## SPICY CHICKEN WITH DICED CARROTS AND GREEN PEPPERS

1½ pounds boneless, skinless
  chicken breasts
1 tablespoon double black soy
  sauce*
1 tablespoon sherry
1 tablespoon cornstarch
1 tablespoon water + ½ cup
  water
2 teaspoons minced garlic

2 teaspoons minced ginger root
2 tablespoons bean sauce
2 teaspoons hot chili paste with
  garlic
1 tablespoon olive oil
¾ cup diced onion
2 cups diced carrot
2 cups diced green pepper

Cut chicken into ½-inch pieces. Place in a medium bowl.

Combine soy sauce and sherry and pour over chicken. Mix until chicken is well covered.

Marinate in refrigerator at least 15 minutes.

In a small bowl, add 1 tablespoon of water to cornstarch and stir into a smooth paste. Stir in remaining water. Set aside.

In a small bowl, combine garlic, ginger, bean sauce, and chili paste and set aside.

In a wok or large skillet, heat olive oil. Sauté chicken and marinade until cooked through. Add 1–2 tablespoons of water to help cook chicken.

Mix in onion, carrots, and green pepper and stir for a few seconds.

Add garlic mixture and stir until chicken and vegetables are well covered.

Mix in cornstarch-water mixture. Let sauce thicken.

Serve over rice.

*6 servings*
*Calories per serving: 146 total; 31 fat; 5 sat-fat*

---

*Available at Asian food stores and some supermarkets.

# SWEDISH CHICKEN MEATBALLS

Suzanne Lieblich took her mother's Swedish meatball recipe, which had been passed down from mother to daughter for generations, and modified it to make it low-fat. Her delicious chicken meatballs can be eaten plain, added to spaghetti sauce or other sauce, made into a meatball sandwich, or reshaped into the fantastic chickenburgers you'll find on page 50. These are meatballs you can enjoy without guilt.

The recipe uses 1 pound of boneless, skinless chicken breasts to make 18 meatballs, but if you want more, just double, triple, or quadruple the ingredients, keeping the proportion of chicken to vegetables and bread the same.

| | |
|---|---|
| 1 carrot, cut into fourths | 1 pound boneless, skinless |
| 1 celery stalk, cut into fourths | chicken breasts |
| ½ red or green pepper, cut into fourths | Dash of salt (optional) |
| 1 small onion, cut into fourths | 2 cans (10¾ oz each) |
| 2 slices whole-wheat bread | chicken broth, defatted |

In a food processor, chop the carrot, celery, pepper, and onion. You should have 2 cups of finely chopped vegetables. Set aside in a small bowl.

Put bread in food processor and process until it becomes fine crumbs. (Don't use commercial bread crumbs.) Set aside in a small bowl.

Cut chicken breasts into thirds and grind in food processor.

In a large bowl, combine ground chicken, vegetables, bread crumbs, and a dash of salt. Form 18 meatballs.

In a soup pot, bring chicken broth to a boil. Add a few meatballs. Cook each one until it is almost completely white before turning. Make sure they are cooked through but not overcooked. Remove to a bowl while you cook remaining meatballs.

You may serve these immediately over spaghetti with the broth as a sauce, use them in a separate sauce, or serve as an appetizer. Or you may refrigerate them in a container with the broth for future use.

*18 meatballs*
*Calories per meatball: 33 total; 3 fat; 1 sat-fat*

## SWEET-SOUR GRILLED CHICKEN

6 boneless, skinless chicken
   breasts
1 cup crushed tomatoes
3 tablespoons sweet orange
   marmalade

¼ cup Dijon mustard
¼ cup lemon juice
1 tablespoon brown sugar
1–3 teaspoons Tabasco sauce
   (optional)

Place chicken in a ceramic or glass container.

Combine remaining ingredients and spoon ¾ cup over chicken. Refrigerate remaining sauce. Marinate chicken in refrigerator for at least 20 minutes; several hours is better.

Preheat the broiler or prepare the grill.

Remove chicken from marinade and place on broiler pan or grill. Spoon excess marinade over breasts and cook for about 10–15 minutes or until cooked through. Heat reserved sauce and spoon over cooked chicken.

*6 servings*
*Calories per serving: 178 total; 13 fat; 4 sat-fat*

# SZECHUAN CHICKEN WITH SWEET RED PEPPER AND PINEAPPLE

NOTE: Try this recipe with a sliced green pepper and no pineapple.

⅓ cup unbleached white flour
Salt to taste (optional)
¼ teaspoon freshly ground black
    pepper
5 boneless, skinless chicken
    breasts
2 tablespoons soy sauce
2 tablespoons dry sherry
1–2 teaspoons chili paste with
    garlic*
1½ tablespoons tomato paste

¼ teaspoon sugar
2 tablespoons cornstarch
2 tablespoons + 1 cup water
1–2 teaspoons chopped ginger
    root
2 green onions, sliced
1 teaspoon olive oil
1 sweet red pepper, sliced
1½ cups pineapple chunks
¼ cup water

Preheat oven to 375°F.

Place flour, salt, and pepper in a plastic bag. Piece by piece, coat chicken by shaking it in the bag.

Arrange floured chicken in one layer in a shallow baking pan and bake for 20–40 minutes or until chicken is cooked through.

Meanwhile, combine soy sauce, sherry, chili paste, tomato paste, and sugar. Set aside.

Combine cornstarch with 2 tablespoons water. Then stir in remaining cup of water. Set aside.

When chicken is cooked, cut into bite-size pieces and set aside.

In a large skillet or wok, sauté ginger and green onions in olive oil for a few seconds.

Remove skillet from heat and mix in soy sauce mixture. Stir in cornstarch-water mixture and return skillet to high heat.

When sauce begins to thicken, add the chicken, red pepper, and pineapple and stir until well coated. If sauce is too thick, add more water, 1 tablespoon at a time.

*5 servings*
*Calories per serving: 203 total; 21 fat; 5 sat-fat*

---

*Available at Asian food stores and some supermarkets.

# TANDOORI CHICKEN

1 clove garlic, minced
½ tablespoon sliced ginger root
2 tablespoons chopped onion
½ teaspoon Dijon mustard
⅛ teaspoon cardamom
⅛ teaspoon coriander
¼ teaspoon salt (optional)

¼ teaspoon freshly ground black pepper
1½ tablespoons fresh lemon juice
¾ cup nonfat yogurt
4 boneless, skinless chicken breasts

Combine all ingredients except chicken (may be done in food processor, mincing garlic and ginger first) and pour over chicken breasts.

Marinate in refrigerator for at least 24 hours.

Place chicken with marinade in a shallow baking pan.

Bake at 375°F for 30–45 minutes or until chicken is fully cooked.

*4 servings*
*Calories per serving: 152 total; 13 fat; 4 sat-fat*

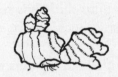

# THAI CHICKEN WITH ASPARAGUS

1 pound asparagus

2 tablespoons cornstarch

2 tablespoons water

1 pound boneless, skinless
   chicken breasts

1 tablespoon olive oil

¼–½ teaspoon red pepper flakes

½ teaspoon caraway seeds

½ teaspoon coriander

½ teaspoon salt (optional)

¼ teaspoon freshly ground black
   pepper

1 tablespoon minced shallot

1 clove garlic, minced

1 can chicken broth (10¾ oz),
   defatted

Snap off and discard the bottoms of asparagus. Cut spears into 1½-inch pieces.

Bring a pot of water to a boil and cook asparagus 3–5 minutes or until tender. Drain, run cool water over asparagus, and set aside.

Mix cornstarch with water until smooth. Set aside.

Cut chicken breasts into bite-size pieces and sauté in oil until cooked through.

While chicken is cooking, combine seasonings, shallot, and garlic (this step is easy to do in a food processor or mini food processor) and mix them together with chicken broth. Add cornstarch mixture. When chicken is cooked through, add seasoned broth. Bring to a boil and let sauce thicken. Lower heat and add asparagus.

*4 servings*
*Calories per serving: 201 total; 42 fat; 8 sat-fat*

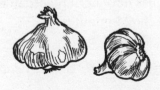

# TORTILLAS CON POLLO

Chicken, yogurt, and rice make this tortilla unusual, low-fat, and, of course, delicious.

### Tomato Sauce

1 clove garlic, minced
⅓ cup chopped onion
1 teaspoon olive oil
1 large can (28 oz) tomatoes,
    drained and chopped

¼ cup chopped green pepper
½ teaspoon cumin seed
½ teaspoon oregano

### Filling

3 cups cooked long-grain rice
1½ cups diced cooked chicken
½–1 teaspoon chili powder

½ teaspoon ground cumin
½ cup nonfat yogurt

8 tortillas*

At least 30 minutes before preparing tortillas, prepare tomato sauce: Cook garlic and onion in olive oil until soft. Add tomatoes, green pepper, cumin seed, and oregano and cook until thick (about 30 minutes).

Preheat oven to 350°F. Grease a shallow baking dish with margarine.

Combine rice, chicken, chili powder, cumin, and yogurt.

Place ½ cup rice mixture in center of each tortilla and roll.

Place seam-side down in baking dish.

When all eight tortillas have been placed in baking dish, cover with tomato sauce and bake for 25 minutes.

*8 servings*
*Calories per serving: 207 total; 16 fat; 1 sat-fat*

---

*Read the label. Packaged tortillas should contain only corn (perhaps some lime) and should *not* contain shortening, fat, salt, or preservatives.

# VEGETABLES, CHICKEN, AND CELLOPHANE NOODLES

2 ounces cellophane noodles*
2 boneless, skinless chicken
   breasts
8 mushrooms (approximately)
2 carrots
1 zucchini
4 green onions

4 leaves Chinese cabbage*
3 cloves garlic, minced
1 tablespoon olive oil
1 tablespoon sesame oil*
3 tablespoons soy sauce
½ teaspoon sugar
½ teaspoon salt, optional

Cover cellophane noodles with warm water and set aside.

Steam chicken breasts in a vegetable steamer. When cooked through (about 10 minutes), cut into bite-size pieces and set aside.

Cut mushrooms into thin slices. Cut carrot and zucchini into julienne strips. Cut green onions into 1-inch pieces. Set aside.

Remove the green part of the Chinese cabbage leaf. Cut into bite-size pieces. Set aside.

Julienne the white part of the leaf. Set aside.

Drain water from cellophane noodles.

Sauté garlic in both oils.

Add vegetables and stir-fry until tender but crisp.

Stir in chicken.

Stir in soy sauce, sugar, salt, and cellophane noodles. Mix to distribute sauce evenly. Serve over rice.

*6 servings*
*Calories per serving: 111 total; 44 fat; 7 sat-fat*

---

*Available at Asian food stores and some supermarkets.

# ~3~
# Turkey

**TURKEY IS THE HEART** of any Thanksgiving dinner, but it makes delicious eating throughout the year. Turkey can be stuffed and roasted and the leftovers made into numerous interesting dishes. Turkey cutlets can replace veal cutlets with no one being the wiser (but everyone being the healthier).

White-meat turkey breast is a must for everyone who wants to consume less fat and who also enjoys eating. One ounce of turkey breast has only 1 calorie of fat!

NOTE: Turkey contains so much protein and so little fat, it tends to cook quickly. Be careful. Overcooking makes turkey tough.

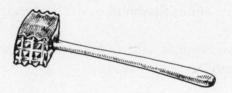

## BASIC TURKEY CUTLETS

Turkey cutlets provide a quick and extremely elegant meal. They can be substituted for exorbitantly expensive veal scaloppine.

1 pound turkey cutlets
½ cup unbleached white flour
1 tablespoon olive oil*

1 tablespoon margarine*
Salt and freshly ground black
    pepper to taste

---

*No fat is used in the second cooking method.

## Two methods to prepare turkey cutlets
## for any veal scaloppine recipe:

**With fat:** Place cutlets between two pieces of wax paper and pound with meat mallet or rolling pin until thin.

Place flour on a plate. Dip each cutlet in flour, coating it on both sides, and place it on a large plate. When the plate is completely covered with one layer of cutlets, cover with a sheet of wax paper to hold the next layer.

Heat olive oil and margarine in a large frying pan or wok.

When very hot (margarine should bubble), place cutlets in frying pan. Do not crowd cutlets.

When the edges turn white, turn cutlets and cook until they are light brown and no longer pink inside. Cutlets cook very quickly. Turn again. Do not overcook or cutlets will be tough.

Remove cutlets to a plate and salt and pepper them liberally.

*Do not clean skillet.* Now you are ready for any scaloppine recipe.

**With no fat added:** If you wish to reduce the total fat content of turkey cutlets (the sat-fat content is already low), instead of sautéing after you pound and flour them, place them on a cast-iron pancake griddle and cook them with no fat. This method works particularly well in the Turkey with Capers recipe.

*4 servings*

| Calories per serving: | Total | Fat | Sat-fat |
|---|---|---|---|
| | 176 | 60 | 12 |
| With no added fat | 124 | 8 | 4 |

## TURKEY BAYOU

This great-tasting dish may also be made with 1¼ pounds of boneless, skinless chicken breasts.

1¼ pounds turkey cutlets

2 teaspoons ground ginger

2 teaspoons sweet paprika

1 teaspoon garlic powder

1 teaspoon ground sage

½ teaspoon onion powder

¾ teaspoon freshly ground black pepper

¼–½ teaspoon cayenne

1 can (10¾ oz) chicken broth, defatted

3 tablespoons cornstarch

½ cup water

1–2 red bell peppers, coarsely chopped

1–2 green peppers, coarsely chopped

2 celery stalks, sliced

1 cup sliced onions

1 tablespoon minced ginger root

3 tablespoons soy sauce

4 cups torn spinach

½ cup water

Cut turkey into bite-size pieces and spread in a single layer on a large plate.

In a small bowl, mix together ginger, paprika, garlic powder, sage, onion powder, black pepper, and cayenne.

Sprinkle 1 tablespoon spice mixture over turkey and rub in. Set aside.

Mix 2 tablespoons of the chicken broth with cornstarch to make a smooth paste. Mix in ½ cup of water and set aside.

Heat a 12-inch heavy skillet (or 10-inch Dutch oven) until hot.

Add turkey. Stir frequently until turkey is almost totally cooked.

Lower heat to medium and add red and green peppers, celery, and onions. Stir well.

Add fresh ginger and remaining spice mixture. Stir well.

Stir in remaining broth and soy sauce. Add cornstarch mixture. Let sauce thicken.

Mix in spinach and ½ cup water.

Serve over rice.

*8 servings*
*Calories per serving: 117 total; 5 fat; 1 sat-fat*

# TURKEY CUTLETS WITH ARTICHOKE-CREAM SAUCE

1 pound turkey cutlets
1 tablespoon margarine
3 tablespoons unbleached white
 flour

1 cup skim milk
1 jar (11½ oz) artichoke hearts,
 packed in water
¼ teaspoon salt (optional)

Prepare cutlets as in master recipe (pages 98–99).

In a medium saucepan, melt margarine. Remove from heat and stir in flour to make a smooth paste.

Slowly stir in skim milk and liquid from artichokes. Add salt. Heat until thick.

Mix in artichoke hearts.

Pour sauce over cutlets and serve.

*5 servings*

| *Calories per serving:* | *Total* | *Fat* | *Sat-fat* |
|---|---|---|---|
|  | 230 | 67 | 15 |
| With no added fat | 188 | 25 | 9 |

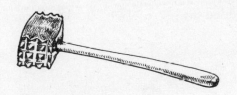

# TURKEY WITH CAPERS

You may sauté turkey cutlets as in the first method for preparing turkey cutlets (page 99), but this takes a lot of fat. Flouring turkey cutlets, then grilling them on a cast-iron pancake griddle with no added fat, as in the second method, produces cutlets that are also tender but have almost no fat calories.

| | |
|---|---|
| 1 pound turkey breast cutlets | 3 tablespoons red wine vinegar |
| 1 teaspoon olive oil | 2 tablespoons Dijon mustard |
| 1 clove garlic, minced | 1 cup chicken broth, strained |
| ¼ cup chopped onion | 2 tablespoons tomato paste |
| 3 tablespoons capers, drained | ⅓ cup chopped parsley |

Prepare turkey cutlets as in master recipe (pages 98–99). Set aside. In a large skillet, sauté garlic and onion in olive oil until soft.

Stir in capers, vinegar, Dijon mustard, chicken broth, and tomato paste. Add parsley.

Add turkey cutlets and mix to cover with sauce.

*4 servings*

| *Calories per serving:* | *Total* | *Fat* | *Sat-fat* |
|---|---|---|---|
| | 227 | 70 | 13 |
| With no added fat | 174 | 18 | 5 |

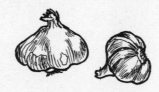

# TURKEY MEXIQUE

A great dish with a chili taste.

1 cup chopped onion
2 teaspoons minced garlic
1 teaspoon olive oil
1–2 tablespoons chili powder
1 tablespoon cumin seed
½ teaspoon salt (optional)
1 tablespoon unbleached white
   flour
1½ cups chicken broth, defatted

3 tablespoons tomato paste
3 cups diced turkey breast, raw
   or cooked
1 green pepper, diced
2–3 cups sliced mushrooms
   (optional)
¼ cup stuffed green olives, sliced
½ cup water

In a large skillet, sauté onion and garlic in olive oil. Add a splash of water and cook until vegetables are soft.

Stir in chili powder, cumin seed, salt, and flour.

Add chicken broth and tomato paste and blend well.

Cook for 5 minutes over low heat.

Stir in turkey, green pepper, mushrooms, and olives and heat through. (If turkey is raw, cook until turkey turns white and is fully cooked.)

If sauce is too thick, add water 2 tablespoons at a time until desired consistency.

Serve over rice.

*6 servings*
*Calories per serving: 146 total; 16 fat; 4 sat-fat*

# TURKEY NIÇOISE

1 pound turkey breast cutlets
¾ cup chopped onion
3 cloves garlic, minced
1 teaspoon olive oil
1½ pounds fresh tomatoes,
　chopped
6 flat anchovies, chopped
½ cup dry vermouth

1 tablespoon capers
8 large black olives, halved
¼–½ teaspoon red pepper flakes
¼ teaspoon thyme
¼ teaspoon basil
¼ teaspoon oregano
Salt to taste (optional)

Prepare turkey cutlets as in master recipe (page 99).

In a large skillet, sauté onion and garlic in 1 teaspoon olive oil until soft. Add a splash of water to help cook the vegetables.

Add tomatoes and anchovies and cook for 10–20 minutes until tomato sauce thickens.

Add vermouth, capers, olives, red pepper flakes, thyme, basil, oregano, and salt to taste, and cook for about 5 minutes until sauce thickens.

Mix turkey cutlets into the sauce and serve.

*6 servings*

| Calories per serving: | Total | Fat | Sat-fat |
|---|---|---|---|
| | 206 | 55 | 11 |
| With no added fat | 171 | 20 | 6 |

# TURKEY WITH SWEET RED PEPPER SAUCE

The sauce takes about an hour to cook but no time to prepare. You may make this tasty dish in advance and refrigerate it.

### Sweet Red Pepper Sauce

2 red peppers, chopped (about 2 cups)

1½ cups sliced tomatoes

1 can chicken broth (10¾ oz), defatted

1 cup dry vermouth

Juice of ½ lemon

¼–½ teaspoon red pepper flakes

Salt to taste (optional)

Freshly ground black pepper to taste

### Garnish

½ cup chopped parsley

Peel of ½ lemon

4 cloves garlic

1 pound turkey cutlets

In a medium (about 8-inch) skillet, combine red peppers, tomatoes, chicken broth, vermouth, lemon juice, red pepper flakes, salt, and black pepper.

Bring to a boil, lower heat to medium, and cook until liquid is reduced and sauce is thick, about 50–60 minutes.

Meanwhile, in a food processor or by hand, chop or mince parsley with lemon peel and garlic. Set aside.

Prepare turkey cutlets as in master recipe (pages 98–99).

Heat red pepper sauce.

Sprinkle parsley mixture over cutlets and cover with sauce.

### 5 servings

| Calories per serving: | Total | Fat | Sat-fat |
|---|---|---|---|
|  | 237 | 48 | 10 |
| With no added fat | 185 | 6 | 3 |

## TURKEY SCALOPPINE LIMONE

| | |
|---|---|
| 1 pound turkey cutlets | ⅓ cup chopped parsley |
| 1 teaspoon margarine | ½ pound mushrooms, sliced |
| ½ cup fresh lemon juice | (optional) |
| 1 teaspoon unbleached white flour | 1 lemon, thinly sliced |

Prepare turkey cutlets as in master recipe (pages 98–99).

Melt margarine in skillet. Add lemon juice.

Sprinkle on flour and blend into mixture. Add cutlets. Stir and turn cutlets until covered with sauce but do not overcook.

Add parsley and mushrooms, stirring until mushrooms are covered with sauce.

Garnish with lemon slices and serve immediately.

*4 servings*

| Calories | Total | Fat | Sat-fat |
|---|---|---|---|
| | 246 | 70 | 14 |
| With no added fat | 194 | 18 | 6 |

## TURKEY SCALOPPINE MARSALA

| | |
|---|---|
| 1 pound turkey cutlets | 2 teaspoons unbleached white flour |
| ½–¾ cup Marsala wine | |
| 1 teaspoon margarine | ½ pound mushrooms, sliced |

Prepare turkey cutlets as in master recipe (pages 98–99).

Add Marsala to pan over high heat. When it begins to boil, add margarine and reduce heat to medium.

Sprinkle on flour and blend.

Add cutlets and stir and turn until covered with sauce.

Add mushrooms and stir until covered with sauce.

*4 servings*

| Calories per serving: | Total | Fat | Sat-fat |
|---|---|---|---|
| | 268 | 70 | 14 |
| With no added fat | 216 | 18 | 6 |

# ~4~
# Fish and Shellfish

**FISH IS AN EXCELLENT CHOICE** for heart-healthy eating. It is a fine source of complete protein. The quality of this protein is about the same as that of red meat. Fish also contains important vitamins and minerals. And, in addition to all this good nutrition, fish contains omega-3 polyunsaturated fats, which have an unusually potent effect in lowering blood triglyceride levels. Fish varies from being extremely low in fat (cod, scallops, haddock, and lobster contain 2 fat calories per ounce; grouper, snapper, and sole contain 3; and monkfish and shrimp, 4) to high (pompano contains 24 fat calories an ounce; Chinook salmon contains 27; Atlantic mackerel, 35; and sablefish, 39).

Fish cooks quickly — within minutes — and may be prepared in a multitude of tasty ways: broiled, baked, poached, oven-fried. Fish may be used as the base for soups, salads, pastas, and stews. Even when prepared most simply to enhance its delicacy, fish is delicious. The key is freshness.

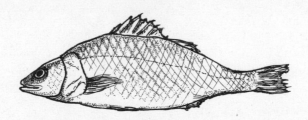

# BLACKENED FISH

This spicy fish will wake up your taste buds. A cool salsa (page 216) enhances this dish.

### Seasoning mix

1 teaspoon paprika
½ teaspoon freshly ground black
   pepper
¼ teaspoon white pepper
¼ teaspoon cayenne

½ teaspoon oregano
½ teaspoon thyme
½ teaspoon basil
½ teaspoon salt (optional)

**1¼ pounds skinned fish fillets**

Preheat broiler.
Combine seasonings on a plate.
Roll each fillet in seasoning mix. Rub mix into both sides. (For a milder version, use less seasoning.)
Broil fillets until cooked through (5–20 minutes depending on thickness of fish).

### 4 servings

| Calories per serving: | Total | Fat | Sat-fat |
|---|---|---|---|
| Sole | 140 | 15 | 5 |
| Swordfish | 170 | 50 | 15 |

## "FRIED" CAJUN CATFISH

You don't have to deep-fry catfish to make it taste delicious. Here's an easy, easy way to oven-bake catfish. For fewer fat calories use a less fatty fish.

½ teaspoon olive oil
½ teaspoon basil
½ teaspoon oregano
½ teaspoon thyme
¼ teaspoon fresh pepper

¼ teaspoon cayenne
½ teaspoon onion powder
½ teaspoon paprika
2 tablespoons cornmeal
4 4-ounce catfish fillets

Preheat oven to 400°F. Grease a baking sheet with the olive oil.

In a small bowl, combine herbs, seasonings, and cornmeal. Spread over a plate large enough to hold a fillet.

Roll fillets one by one in spice mixture until well covered and place in one layer on baking sheet.

Bake for 15–20 minutes until fillets are golden brown and flake easily.

*4 servings*
*Calories per serving: 152 total; 50 fat; 12 sat-fat*

## DILL FISH

1½ pounds fish fillets (flounder, sole, turbot, etc.)
¼ cup fresh lime juice
1 teaspoon dillweed

1 clove garlic, minced
Salt and freshly ground black pepper to taste

Preheat oven to 350°F.

Squeeze lime juice over fillets and marinate for at least 30 minutes in refrigerator.

Grease a shallow baking pan with margarine.

Place fillets in baking pan and sprinkle with dill, garlic, salt, and pepper.

Bake for 5–10 minutes or until fish flakes easily.

*6 servings*
*Calories per serving: 115 total; 12 fat; 4 sat-fat*

## CURRY FISH

A simple but impressive dish, which tastes as good as it looks. Fun for company.

| | |
|---|---|
| 1 pound any white fish fillets | Raisins |
| Salt to taste | Peanuts |
| 2 teaspoons olive oil | Crushed pineapple |
| ½–1 tablespoon curry powder | Scallions |
| 2½ cups cooked long-grain rice | Chutney |
| 2 hard-boiled egg whites, chopped | |

Preheat oven to 425°F. Grease a baking dish with margarine.

Place fillets in baking dish, salt lightly, and bake for 20 minutes.

Flake the fish. (If you wish to serve it later, you can refrigerate the fish now.)

Heat olive oil in a large skillet and mix in curry powder.

Add fish and stir until it is covered with curry sauce.

Mix cooked rice and fish together gently.

Place egg whites, raisins, peanuts, crushed pineapple, scallions, and chutney in small dishes and pass with main dish.

*4 servings*

| *Calories per serving:* | Total | Fat | Sat-fat |
|---|---|---|---|
| Without condiments | 283 | 28 | 5 |
| With teaspoon of each | 349 | 41 | 7 |

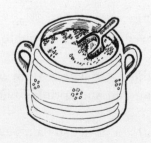

# FLOUNDER FILLETS STUFFED
# WITH FENNEL RICE

Raw fennel, or *finocchio*, as the Italians call it, tastes of licorice or anise. The taste of cooked fennel is more subtle and sweet. Cook sliced fennel bulb with margarine and water to cover for a delicious vegetable dish. You may substitute celery in this recipe, but try to find fennel at your grocery store or an Italian market for a more unusual dish.

⅓ cup sliced fennel stalks

⅓ cup sliced mushrooms

1 teaspoon fennel seeds

1 teaspoon olive oil

1½ cups cooked long-grain rice

2 tablespoons margarine

3 tablespoons fresh lemon juice

8 4-ounce flounder fillets

Preheat oven to 375°F. Grease a shallow baking pan with margarine.

In a medium skillet, sauté fennel and mushrooms in olive oil until just tender.

Add fennel seeds and cooked rice. Stir for a minute and set aside.

Melt 2 tablespoons margarine in a small saucepan. Add lemon juice and set aside.

Lay out fillets on waxed paper.

Place several tablespoons of rice mixture in middle of each fillet.

Roll up fillets and place them seam-side down in baking dish. (The sides may barely reach each other, but that is okay.)

Pour margarine-lemon mixture over fish and bake for about 20 minutes or until fillets flake easily. (Measure thickness of rolled fish and allow 10 minutes per inch.)

If you have any rice mixture left over, reheat and serve with fish.

*8 servings*
*Calories per serving: 150 total; 28 fat; 6 sat-fat*

# FENNEL FISH

1¼ pounds thick fish fillets, such
   as grouper
1 tablespoon olive oil

3 tablespoons fennel seed
2 tablespoons water

Cut fish crosswise into ½-inch-thick slices. Set aside.

Pour oil into a skillet large enough to hold fish pieces in one layer. Add fennel and sauté for a few seconds.

Add fish. Let cook for about 2 minutes on medium heat.

Add 1 tablespoon of the water and cover skillet. In about 2 more minutes, add the second tablespoon of water and replace cover. Steam the fish until it is cooked through.

Serve immediately.

*4 servings*
*Calories per serving: 134 total; 42 fat; 4 sat-fat*

# BROILED GINGER FISH

1 cup flour
1 teaspoon salt (optional)
½ teaspoon freshly ground black
   pepper
4 six-ounce fish fillets (monkfish,
   haddock, etc.)

2 teaspoons margarine
4 teaspoons diced ginger root
Lemon slices to cover fillets

Set oven to broil and grease broiler pan with oil.

Combine flour, salt, and pepper on a large plate.

Dredge fillets in flour, covering both sides.

Dot fillets with margarine, sprinkle with ginger, and cover with lemon slices.

Broil for 5–15 minutes or until fish flakes easily.

*4 servings*
*Calories per serving: 194 total; 35 fat; 4 sat-fat*

## GREEN AND RED PEPPER FISH

4 green onions, chopped
1 medium onion, chopped
1 green pepper, roughly chopped
1 red pepper, roughly chopped
1 tablespoon minced garlic
½ teaspoon olive oil
1 tablespoon chili powder
2 cups tomato sauce (15-oz can)

½–1 teaspoon freshly ground
  black pepper
¼–½ teaspoon cayenne pepper
½ teaspoon sugar
½ cup vermouth
1 pound mild, low-fat fish (or
  shrimp), cut into bite-size
  pieces

In a large skillet, sauté onions, red and green peppers, and garlic in the oil. Add a splash of water and cook vegetables until tender.

Stir in chili powder. Add tomato sauce, black pepper, cayenne, sugar, and vermouth.

Add fish and cook until fish is opaque.

*6 servings*
*Calories per serving: 148 total; 11 fat; 3 sat-fat*

## FISH WITH MUSHROOM SAUCE

8 fillets (6 oz each) pollack,
  monkfish, or other white fish

Make mushroom sauce (see page 118).
Preheat oven to 350°F. Grease a shallow baking pan with margarine.
Place fish in baking pan.
Bake for 5–10 minutes or until fish is opaque and flakes easily.
Spoon mushroom sauce over fish and serve.

*8 servings*
*Calories per serving: 254 total; 40 fat; 8 sat-fat*

# MARINATED FISH STEAKS

1½ pounds fish steaks
  (swordfish, cod, halibut, etc.)
2 tablespoons ketchup
1 tablespoon fresh lemon juice
1 clove garlic, minced
1 teaspoon oregano

½ teaspoon salt (optional)
1 teaspoon olive oil
¼ cup orange juice
¼ cup dry vermouth
¼ cup chopped parsley

Place steaks in a shallow casserole dish.

Combine ketchup, lemon juice, garlic, oregano, salt, olive oil, orange juice, vermouth, and parsley and pour over fish. Marinate several hours or overnight in refrigerator.

Preheat broiler and grease broiler pan with oil.

Broil fish for 5–15 minutes or until it flakes easily.

Heat marinade and spoon over fish.

*4 servings*

| Calories per serving: | Total | Fat | Sat-fat |
|---|---|---|---|
| Swordfish | 241 | 70 | 17 |
| Cod | 175 | 22 | 1 |
| Halibut | 240 | 42 | 7 |

# FISH BAKED IN OLIVE, CHILI PEPPER, AND TOMATO SAUCE

¾ cup chopped onion

2 cloves garlic, minced

1 teaspoon olive oil

1 tablespoon cornstarch

1 can (16 oz) tomatoes, chopped, juice reserved

⅓ cup sliced stuffed green olives

1 teaspoon chopped red or green chili pepper

1½ pounds flounder fillets (or other mild fish)

Salt to taste (optional)

1 tablespoon fresh lemon juice

Preheat oven to 375°F.

In a medium skillet, sauté onion and garlic in olive oil. Add a splash of water and cook until soft.

Mix in cornstarch.

Add tomatoes and their juice and mix until well blended.

Cook over medium-high heat until sauce thickens.

Stir in olives and chili pepper.

Spoon half the sauce into a baking pan large enough to hold fillets in one layer. Place fillets over sauce.

Salt fillets and sprinkle with lemon juice.

Cover fillets with remaining sauce and bake for 10 minutes or until they flake easily.

*6 servings*
*Calories per serving: 150 total; 18 fat; 5 sat-fat*

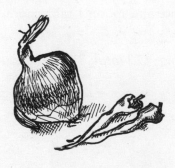

# BROILED MONKFISH WITH ORANGE SAUCE

Very special and delicious. Skim milk makes a great cream sauce. (And look at the difference in fat calories per cup: 0 for a cup of skim milk versus 665 for a cup of light cream.)

| | |
|---|---|
| 1 tablespoon margarine | ¼ cup flour |
| 2 tablespoons unbleached white flour | ½ teaspoon salt (optional) |
| ¼ cup orange juice | ¼ teaspoon freshly ground black pepper |
| ¾ cup skim milk | 1½ pounds monkfish fillets (or any white fish fillets) |
| Grated rind of 1 orange | |
| 1 green onion, sliced | 2 teaspoons margarine |
| ¼ teaspoon salt (optional) | |

Preheat broiler and grease broiler pan with oil.

Melt margarine in a small saucepan. Remove from heat and mix in 2 tablespoons flour to make a smooth paste.

Mix in orange juice and skim milk, stirring until smooth.

Cook over medium heat until sauce thickens, stirring constantly.

Stir in 2 tablespoons grated orange rind, green onion, and salt and set aside.

Combine ¼ cup flour, salt, and pepper and place on large plate.

Dredge fillets in flour so both sides are coated.

Lay fillets on broiler pan and dot with 2 teaspoons margarine.

Sprinkle remaining orange rind on fillets (grate more if needed).

Broil for 5–15 minutes, depending on thickness of fish, or until fish flakes easily.

Reheat orange sauce and spoon 1 tablespoon over each serving.

*6 servings*
*Calories per serving: 179 total; 37 fat; 12 sat-fat*

# ORIENTAL FISH KEBABS

1¼ pounds swordfish steaks
½ cup fresh lime juice
1 tablespoon soy sauce
1 tablespoon brown sugar
2 cloves garlic, minced
2 tablespoons sliced green onion

1 medium onion, cut into
   eighths
1 green pepper, cut into 1½-inch
   pieces
8 cherry tomatoes

Cut fish into 1½-inch cubes.

Combine lime juice, soy sauce, brown sugar, garlic, and green onion and pour over fish. Marinate for at least 2 hours in refrigerator.

Arrange fish, onion chunks, green pepper, and tomatoes on skewers. Rotate skewers in marinade to cover vegetables and let sit for several minutes so the vegetables can absorb the flavor.

Broil for 10 minutes per inch of thickness of fish or until it flakes easily.

Heat remaining marinade and spoon over fish.

*4 servings*
*Calories per serving: 243 total; 51 fat; 10 sat-fat*

## PHYLLO-WRAPPED FISH
## AND MUSHROOM SAUCE

Fish wrapped in phyllo dough is an elegant company dish. If you want a simpler (as in less work) dish, just ignore the phyllo part of the recipe. The fish with mushroom sauce is still luscious.

NOTE: If you are using phyllo dough, the directions on the box usually recommend that you thaw it in the refrigerator overnight and 2–3 hours at room temperature before you use it.

| | |
|---|---|
| 8 fillets (6 oz each) pollack, monkfish, or other white fish | 1 pound phyllo leaves |
| Salt and freshly ground black pepper | 2 tablespoons melted margarine |

### Mushroom Sauce

| | |
|---|---|
| 2 tablespoons margarine | ¼ teaspoon salt |
| ¼ cup unbleached white flour | ⅛ teaspoon freshly ground black pepper |
| 3 cups sliced mushrooms | |
| ¼ cup dry sherry | Grated nutmeg to taste |
| 1¼ cups skim milk | |

### The Fish

Preheat oven to 350°F. Grease a baking sheet with margarine.

Check fillets for small bones and remove them.

Lightly salt and pepper fish.

Unroll thawed phyllo dough and cover it with plastic wrap or a towel to keep it from drying out and becoming brittle.

Place one sheet of phyllo on the counter with a narrow end toward you. Brush with melted margarine. Cover with a second sheet of phyllo and brush it with melted margarine. Repeat process for third sheet.

Place fillet on the phyllo edge nearest you. (If fillet is long and narrow, you may have to fold the fillet in half.) Fold left side, then right side of phyllo over fillet and roll it up.

Place seam-side down on baking sheet.

Wrap each fillet in phyllo dough and place on baking sheet.

Bake for 20 minutes. Make a small slit in phyllo to see if fish is done. Bake until fish flakes easily and is opaque.

While fish is baking, make mushroom sauce.

### The Mushroom Sauce

In a medium saucepan, melt margarine.

Lower heat and mix in flour. Remove pan from heat.

In a medium skillet, cook mushrooms in sherry until all but ¼ cup liquid is evaporated. Drain liquid from mushrooms and set it aside. Set mushrooms aside.

In a small saucepan, heat milk until steaming but *not boiling*. Slowly pour milk into flour mixture, blending until sauce is smooth. Stir in mushroom liquid.

Return saucepan to burner and slowly heat sauce to boiling.

Add mushrooms, salt, pepper, and nutmeg to thickened sauce.

Serve over phyllo-wrapped fish.

*8 servings*

| *Calories per serving:* | *Total* | *Fat* | *Sat-fat* |
|---|---|---|---|
| With mushroom sauce | 318 | 70 | 15 |
| Without mushroom sauce | 253 | 48 | 5 |

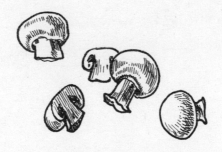

# FISH WITH PEPPERCORNS, THYME, AND MUSTARD

¼–½ teaspoon black
  peppercorns
4 teaspoons Dijon mustard
1 teaspoon thyme

2 tablespoons vermouth
½ teaspoon olive oil
1 pound fish fillets (sole,
  flounder, etc.)

Preheat oven to 450°F. Use margarine to grease shallow glass casserole or baking pan large enough to hold fish.

Crush peppercorns coarsely in food processor or with mortar and pestle.

Combine peppercorns with mustard, thyme, vermouth, and oil.

Make several diagonal slashes across fillets.

Place fish in baking pan and spread mustard mixture over it.

Bake for 5–20 minutes, or until fish flakes easily.

*3 servings*
*Calories per serving: 70 total; 23 fat; 5 sat-fat*

# FISH STEAKS WITH CUCUMBER-GRAPE SAUCE

¼ cup nonfat yogurt
1½ tablespoons low-fat
   mayonnaise
½ tablespoon fresh lemon juice
¼ cup grated cucumber

1 cup seedless grapes
6 fish steaks (4 oz each)
1 tablespoon margarine
3 tablespoons fresh lemon juice

Preheat broiler and grease broiler pan.
Combine yogurt, mayonnaise, lemon juice, cucumber, and grapes.
Set aside.
Place fish steaks on broiler pan.
Melt margarine and combine it with lemon juice.
Baste fish with lemon-margarine sauce.
Broil 3–5 minutes, turn fish, and baste again.
Broil 3–5 minutes more, or until fish flakes easily.
Spoon cucumber-grape sauce over fish and serve.

*6 servings*

| Calories per serving: | Total | Fat | Sat-fat |
|---|---|---|---|
| Monkfish | 129 | 33 | 7 |
| Salmon* | 205 | 80 | 15 |
| Tuna | 209 | 65 | 15 |

*Salmon varies greatly in total calories and sat-fat calories depending on the variety.
This will affect the total calories per serving.

## SALMON SOUFFLÉ

1 can (8 oz) salmon
1 cup skim milk
1 cup fine bread crumbs made
   from 2 slices whole-wheat
   bread

3 egg whites

Preheat oven to 350°F. Grease a small casserole with margarine.

Prepare salmon by carefully rinsing it with water and removing any bones. Set aside.

Heat skim milk and bread crumbs slowly in a double boiler until thick.

Meanwhile, whip egg whites until stiff but not dry. Set aside.

Flake salmon with a fork and add it to the thickened milk mixture. Remove from heat.

Fold salmon mixture into egg whites.

Pour into casserole and bake for 30 minutes.

*4 servings*
*Calories per serving: 149 total; 32 fat; 9 sat-fat*

# SALMON SUBLIME

The combination of honey, grainy mustard, and soy sauce makes such a sweet crust that Ron says eating this dish is like eating candy.

4 tablespoons grainy Dijon
  mustard*
4 tablespoons honey

2 teaspoons soy sauce
1 pound salmon steaks or fillets

Combine the mustard, honey, and soy sauce.

Place the steaks or fillets in a glass or ceramic container. Spread ¼ cup of the sauce over them and marinate in refrigerator for several hours. Refrigerate remaining sauce.

Preheat broiler for about 10 minutes.

Place a sheet of aluminum foil on broiler pan. Remove fillets from container and place on foil. Cut diagonal slits every 1–2 inches across each fillet. Pour excess marinade over fillets.

Spread reserved sauce over them.

Broil about 3 inches from heating coil for 10–15 minutes, checking after 10 minutes. Fish is done when it is opaque and flakes easily.

*4 servings*
*Calories per serving: 307 total; 64 fat; 12 sat-fat*

*We use Maille L'Ancienne Dijon Mustard. Choose a Dijon mustard that is full of seeds.

## SHANGHAI FISH

1½ pounds white fish fillets
2 tablespoons soy sauce
1 clove garlic, minced

2 tablespoons dry sherry
3 green onions, sliced
1 tablespoon hoisin sauce*

Marinate fish in soy sauce, garlic, sherry, green onions, and hoisin sauce for several hours in refrigerator.

Broil for 5–10 minutes or until fish flakes easily and is opaque.

Heat marinade to boiling and serve over fish.

*6 servings*
*Calories per serving: 117 total; 12 fat; 4 sat-fat*

## FISH IN WINE SAUCE

This delicate fish dish takes no time to make.

¾ pound white fish fillets, such
  as flounder or sole
¼–½ cup white wine or
  vermouth

3 tablespoons minced shallots
Freshly ground black pepper to
  taste

Preheat oven to 400°F. Place the fillets in one layer in a shallow baking pan and pour wine over them. The wine should *not* cover them.

Sprinkle shallots over fish.

Depending on thickness of fish, bake for 5–20 minutes, or until it flakes easily.

Sprinkle liberally with pepper and serve.

*3 servings*
*Calories per serving: 119 total; 12 fat; 4 sat-fat*

---

*Available at Asian food stores and some supermarkets.

## SOUTHWESTERN BROILED FISH FILLETS

This is a quick and easy dish to prepare. You can use any mild fish. Here we use flounder, which has about 3 fat calories per ounce. All the fat in the recipe comes from the fish, so you can keep the fat calories low by choosing a low-fat fish.

| | |
|---|---|
| ¼ cup cilantro | 1 tablespoon soy sauce |
| 1 clove garlic | 2 tablespoons fresh lime juice |
| ¼ cup onion, chopped | 1 medium tomato |
| ½ cup red pepper, chopped | 4 fish fillets (about 6 oz each) |

In a blender or food processor, coarsely blend all ingredients except fillets.

Place fillets in a glass or ceramic container. Pour ½ cup of sauce over fillets and marinate in refrigerator for several hours. Refrigerate remaining sauce.

When ready to cook, preheat broiler for about 10 minutes.

Place a sheet of aluminum foil on broiler pan. Remove fillets from container and place on foil. Cut diagonal slits every 1–2 inches across each one. The fillets should still be covered with some marinade.

Broil for 10 minutes, checking after 5 minutes. Fillets are done when they are opaque and flake easily with a fork.

While the fish is cooking, remove sauce from refrigerator and heat in a small saucepan.

Spoon sauce over each fillet and serve.

*4 servings*
*Calories per serving: 168 total; 18 fat; 6 sat-fat*

# Shrimp and Scallops

Both shrimp and scallops are low-fat gems. They take only 3–5 minutes to cook, may be added to innumerable sauces with no fuss or bother, are extremely low in fat (scallops have 2 fat calories per ounce; shrimp have 4), and are delicious.

You may have been told to avoid shrimp because it is higher in cholesterol than other shellfish. Don't worry. Shrimp contains only slightly more cholesterol than other meats but is extremely low in saturated fat. It also contains risk-reducing omega-3 polyunsaturated fats. We recommend that you eat as much shrimp as you can afford unless you are wealthy or a shrimp fisherman.

## SHRIMP WITH ARTICHOKES AND TOMATOES

¾ pound spaghetti*
1 can (15 oz) artichoke hearts in
   water
4 medium fresh tomatoes
2 teaspoons olive oil
4 cloves garlic, thinly sliced

1 pound shrimp, peeled and
   deveined
1 tablespoon lemon juice
1½ cups clam juice
½ teaspoon basil
½ teaspoon red pepper flakes

Prepare spaghetti according to package directions. Drain and cool on a cookie sheet.

Meanwhile, drain artichoke hearts and cut into fourths. Set aside.

Cut tomatoes into bite-size pieces and set aside.

In a large skillet, sauté garlic in olive oil until fragrant. Add shrimp and stir until cooked. It will turn pink.

Add artichokes and tomatoes and cook for a few moments.

Add lemon juice, clam juice, basil, and pepper flakes.

Divide spaghetti among six bowls and top with shrimp sauce.

*6 servings*
*Calories per serving: 320 total; 34 fat; 4 sat-fat*

---

*If you are cooking for big eaters, you might want to use the whole pound.

## SHRIMP OR SCALLOPS CARIBBEAN

¼ cup sugar
2 tablespoons cornstarch
⅛ teaspoon salt (optional)
½ cup orange juice
⅓ cup white vinegar
½ cup water
1 pound shrimp, shelled and
    deveined, or bay scallops

2 teaspoons grated orange rind
½ pound mushrooms, sliced
1 medium orange, peeled and
    cut into bite-size pieces
¼ pound snow peas
¼ cup sliced green onions

In a large skillet, combine sugar, cornstarch, and salt. Slowly stir in orange juice, vinegar, and water.

Stir constantly over medium heat until mixture thickens.

Add shrimp or scallops and orange rind.

When shellfish is cooked through (5–10 minutes), add mushrooms, orange pieces, snow peas, and green onions.

Serve over rice.

*6 servings*

| Calories per serving: | Total | Fat | Sat-fat |
|---|---|---|---|
| Shrimp | 156 | 11 | 3 |
| Scallops | 143 | 5 | 0 |

## HONEY-CURRY SCALLOPS

2 tablespoons honey
½–1 teaspoon curry powder
2 tablespoons Dijon mustard

1 teaspoon fresh lemon juice
1 pound sea scallops

Preheat broiler.

Mix honey, curry powder, Dijon mustard, and lemon juice in a medium bowl. Add scallops and mix until they are well coated with sauce.

Lay scallops on broiler pan and place pan about 5 inches from source of heat. Broil for 5–10 minutes or until scallops are no longer pink inside. Don't overcook or scallops will be rubbery.

*4 servings (about 5 scallops each)*
*Calories per serving: 140 total; 8 fat; 0 sat-fat*

## SHRIMP OR SCALLOPS CREOLE

2 green peppers, chopped
1 cup chopped onion
2 cloves garlic, minced
2 teaspoons olive oil
1 teaspoon brown sugar
¼ teaspoon freshly ground black
   pepper
1 teaspoon thyme
¼ teaspoon cayenne pepper
1 bay leaf

½ teaspoon salt (optional)
2 large cans (28 oz each)
   tomatoes, drained, juiced,
   and chopped
½ cup sliced celery
1½ cups sliced mushrooms
3 tablespoons chopped parsley
1 pound shrimp, shelled and
   deveined, or scallops

Sauté green peppers, onion, and garlic in olive oil. Add a splash of water and cook vegetables until soft.

Add brown sugar, pepper, thyme, cayenne pepper, bay leaf, and salt and stir well.

Stir in tomatoes and cook over low heat for 30 minutes or until sauce is thick.

Add celery and mushrooms and cook for a few minutes more.

Mix in parsley and shrimp or scallops and cook for 5–10 minutes or until shellfish is cooked through.

Serve immediately so shellfish will not overcook.

Serve over rice.

*6 servings*

| Calories per serving: | Total | Fat | Sat-fat |
|---|---|---|---|
| Shrimp | 177 | 24 | 5 |
| Scallops | 163 | 18 | 2 |

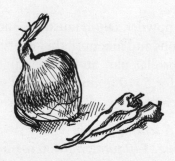

## SHRIMP OR SCALLOP CURRY

Delight your guests or family with this unusual curry. The apples and lime create a unique combination of sweet and sour tastes.

1 cup chopped onion
1 apple, peeled, cored, and diced
2 cloves garlic, minced
1–3 teaspoons curry powder
1 tablespoon olive oil
¼ cup unbleached white flour
½ teaspoon salt (optional)
¼ teaspoon cardamom
¼ teaspoon freshly ground black pepper

1 can chicken broth (10¾ oz), defatted
1 tablespoon fresh lime juice
1¼ pounds shrimp, shelled and deveined, or bay scallops
1 cup sliced mushrooms
10–15 snow peas (optional)
½–1 cup water

In a large skillet, sauté onion, apple, garlic, and curry powder in olive oil until tender.

Remove skillet from heat and blend in flour, salt, cardamom, and pepper.

Stir in chicken broth and lime juice until curry sauce is well blended.

Bring curry sauce to a boil, reduce heat, and simmer, uncovered, for about 5 minutes. Stir occasionally.

Meanwhile, place scallops or shrimp in a pot of boiling water and cook until just tender (5–10 minutes). Drain and set aside.

When curry sauce is finished cooking, add shellfish, mushrooms, and snow peas. If sauce is too thick, add water, ¼ cup at a time until desired consistency is achieved. Serve curry over rice.

*6 servings*

| Calories per serving: | Total | Fat | Sat-fat |
|---|---|---|---|
| Shrimp | 181 | 33 | 6 |
| Scallops | 164 | 27 | 3 |

## SHRIMP WITH GREEN PEPPERS

1 pound shrimp, shelled and
  deveined
2 tablespoons soy sauce
2 tablespoons dry sherry
1–2 teaspoons chili paste with
  garlic*
2 tablespoons tomato paste
½ teaspoon sugar

1 tablespoon cornstarch
2 tablespoons + 1 cup water
1–2 teaspoons chopped ginger
  root
2 green onions, sliced
2 teaspoons olive oil
1 large green pepper, sliced
¼ cup water

Put shrimp in a pot of boiling water and cook for 2–5 minutes or until just cooked. Drain and set aside. (Shrimp may be made a day in advance and refrigerated.)

Combine soy sauce, sherry, chili paste, tomato paste, and sugar. Set aside.

Combine cornstarch with 2 tablespoons water. Then stir in 1 cup water. Set aside.

In a large skillet or wok, sauté ginger and green onions in olive oil for a few seconds.

Remove skillet from heat and stir in soy sauce and cornstarch mixtures. Return skillet to high heat. When sauce begins to thicken, mix in cooked shrimp and green pepper until well coated. If sauce is too thick, add more water, 1 tablespoon at a time.

*4 servings*
*Calories per serving: 174 total; 36 fat; 6 sat-fat*

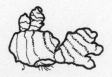

---

*Available at Asian food stores and some supermarkets.

## SPICY SHRIMP LOUISIANA

This dish also tastes great with bite-size pieces of chicken instead of shrimp.

1–1¼ pounds shrimp
¼ teaspoon ground white pepper
⅛ teaspoon freshly ground black
  pepper
¼ teaspoon cayenne pepper
½ teaspoon basil
¼ teaspoon thyme
¼ teaspoon salt (optional)
¼ cup water
¼ cup unbleached white flour

2 teaspoons olive oil
½ cup chopped onion
1 green pepper, chopped
2 stalks celery, chopped
2 cloves garlic, minced
1 can (10¾ oz) chicken broth,
  defatted
1 tablespoon tomato paste
¼ cup chopped green onions

Shell, devein, and clean shrimp. Cook in boiling water for about 3 minutes. Drain and set shrimp aside.

Combine white, black, and cayenne pepper, basil, thyme, and salt. Set aside.

Slowly add water to flour and mix into a paste. Set aside.

Heat oil in wok or large frying pan until hot.

Stir in onion, green pepper, celery, and garlic and cook until soft.

Mix in spice mixture.

Stir in broth and tomato paste.

Stir in flour mixture and cook until sauce thickens.

Add shrimp and green onions and serve over rice.

*6 servings*
*Calories per serving: 88 total; 28 fat; 2 sat-fat*

## SCALLOPS PROVENÇAL

It takes only about 15 minutes and very little effort to create this delightful combination of colors, textures, and tastes.

1 pound bay scallops
¼ cup unbleached white flour
3 cloves garlic, minced
1 tablespoon olive oil

2 cups snow peas (about ½ pound)
2 cups sliced red pepper
1 cup sliced mushrooms

Rinse scallops, dry with a paper towel, and roll in flour.

In a wok or large skillet, sauté scallops and garlic in olive oil until tender (about 5–10 minutes). Add a splash or two of water to help cook scallops.

Add snow peas, red peppers, and mushrooms and mix until heated through.

Serve over rice.

*5 servings*
*Calories per serving: 190 total; 30 fat; 5 sat-fat*

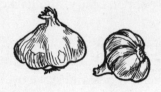

## SWEET AND SOUR SHRIMP

1 pound shrimp
2 tablespoons brown sugar
4 tablespoons white vinegar
¼ cup tomato sauce
¼ cup water
2 teaspoons cornstarch
2 teaspoons soy sauce
2 cloves garlic, minced or pressed

2 teaspoons ginger root, minced
2 large carrots
3 green onions
¾ cup sliced onion
1 teaspoon olive oil
4 tablespoons water
1 red pepper, sliced
1 green pepper, sliced

Peel and devein shrimp. Set aside.

Combine brown sugar, vinegar, tomato sauce, water, cornstarch, soy sauce, garlic, and ginger. Set aside.

Lay both carrots on cutting board and slice each lengthwise at ⅛-inch intervals. Cut these strips into pieces 1½–2 inches long. You should have about 2 cups of strips.

Slice green onions in half and cut into 1-inch pieces. Set aside.

In a wok or large skillet, sauté carrots and onion in olive oil. Mix for a few seconds.

Add 1 tablespoon water and mix for a minute or two. Add 3 more tablespoons water and cover the pan. Cook for a minute or two.

Mix in shrimp, peppers, and green onions. Add sauce. Cover to let steam cook shrimp.

Uncover occasionally to stir shrimp. Add 1 tablespoon water. Cook until shrimp have changed color and are opaque.

*5 servings*
*Calories per serving: 167 total; 21 fat; 4 sat-fat*

# ~5~
# Vegetables

**HOORAY FOR VEGETABLES!** Vegetables provide meals with texture, color, dietary fiber, vitamins, and minerals. They score high in a cancer-prevention eating plan as well as a heart-healthy eating plan. And they are delicious! They fill you up without filling you out.

One of the best ways to cook vegetables is also the easiest. Cook fresh vegetables in a steamer until they are just tender (a few minutes at most). For a nonfat treat, sprinkle on vinegar or minced garlic. Steaming minimizes loss of vitamins. It also brings out the unique taste of each vegetable.

In addition to steaming, vegetables may be prepared in a variety of enticing ways, as you will find in the recipes below.

## ITALIAN MIXED VEGETABLES

1 clove garlic, minced
1 onion, sliced
2 teaspoons olive oil
3 cups combined red and/or
    yellow and/or green peppers,
    sliced

2 zucchini, sliced (about 2 cups)
Salt to taste
1 teaspoon thyme, oregano, or
    basil, or combination

In a large skillet, sauté garlic and onion in olive oil. Add a splash of water and cook vegetables until tender.

Stir in peppers, zucchini, salt, and herbs.

Cover. Cook until tender.

*8 servings*
*Calories per serving: 27 total; 10 fat; 1 sat-fat*

# INDIAN VEGETABLES

Indian Vegetables is one of our all-time favorite recipes. This large pot of colorful, tasty vegetables may be eaten warm or cold. Try it as a main dish served over rice.

2 teaspoons olive oil
1 teaspoon black mustard seeds*
3 cloves garlic, chopped
1 medium onion, chopped
1 green pepper, chopped
2–3 potatoes, peeled and cubed
1 small eggplant, peeled and
   cubed
1½ teaspoons turmeric
1 teaspoon salt (optional)
¼ cup water
1 teaspoon cumin
1 teaspoon coriander

1 teaspoon garam masala*
Any vegetables, for example:
   1 head broccoli, cut into
      flowerets (about 3 cups)
   1 cup or more cauliflower
      flowerets
   6 carrots, sliced
   1 cup or more green beans,
      cut in half
   1 cup sliced celery
   1 zucchini, sliced
1 cup water

In a large pot, heat olive oil and add black mustard seeds.

When the mustard seeds begin to pop, add garlic, onion, and green pepper and cook until soft.

Stir in potatoes and eggplant.

Add turmeric and salt and mix until vegetables are covered with turmeric sauce.

Add ¼ cup water, reduce heat to low, cover pot, and cook for 10 minutes.

Stir in cumin, coriander, garam masala, and vegetables.

Add 1 cup water and increase heat to medium.

After 10 minutes, lower heat and cook until vegetables are tender.

*12 servings*
*Calories per serving: 72 total; 7 fat; 1 sat-fat*

---

*Available at Indian or Mideastern food stores.

## LISA'S VEGETABLE STEW

This is one of many wonderful dishes created by our son Dan's friend Lisa Eisen.

¾ cup chopped onion
5–6 cloves garlic, minced
1 teaspoon olive oil
1 large can (28 oz) tomatoes
3–4 teaspoons curry powder

1 can chickpeas, drained
1 butternut squash (about 1 lb), peeled, seeded, and cubed
2–3 medium potatoes, peeled and cubed

Sauté onion and garlic in olive oil until soft.

Add tomatoes and their juice. Mash tomatoes with a stirring spoon. Stir in curry powder.

Add chickpeas, squash, and potatoes.

Turn down heat and simmer for 1 hour or until vegetables are tender. Add water if stew gets too dry.

*14 half-cup servings*
*Calories per serving: 74 total; 7 fat; 1 sat-fat*

# MURIEL'S CHINESE VEGETABLES

2 ounces cellophane noodles*
3 cups broccoli flowerets (about
   1 head)
2 cups cauliflower flowerets
2 cloves garlic, minced
1 red pepper, sliced

1 teaspoon olive oil
1 teaspoon sesame oil
2 tablespoons dry white wine or
   vermouth
1 teaspoon five-spice powder*
2 tablespoons soy sauce

Pour boiling water over cellophane noodles and let them soak for 15–30 minutes.

Steam broccoli and cauliflower in steamer until just tender. Set aside.

Sauté garlic and red pepper in oils for a few seconds.

Mix in broccoli and cauliflower.

Stir in wine and five-spice powder.

Drain cellophane noodles and stir into vegetables.

Stir in soy sauce until vegetables are well coated with sauce.

*9 servings*
*Calories per serving: 54 total; 9 fat; 1 sat-fat*

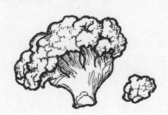

*Available in Asian food stores and some supermarkets.

# RATATOUILLE

Add eggplant, bay leaf, and tomatoes to Italian mixed vegetables and you have a French dish — ratatouille.

2 cloves garlic, minced
1 onion, sliced
2 teaspoons olive oil
3 cups combined red and/or yellow and/or green peppers, sliced
2 zucchini, sliced (about 2 cups)
4 fresh tomatoes, cubed, or 1 large can (28 oz) Italian plum tomatoes, drained

Salt to taste
1 bay leaf
1 teaspoon dried basil or 2 tablespoons fresh basil, chopped
1 small eggplant, cubed and steamed (about 2 cups)*

Sauté garlic and onion in olive oil in a medium-large casserole.

Add peppers, zucchini, tomatoes, salt, bay leaf, and basil.

Cover and simmer until vegetables are tender (about 15–20 minutes).

Add steamed eggplant and cook for 5 minutes more.

*10 servings*
*Calories per serving: 32 total; 8 fat; 2 sat-fat*

---

*See page 148 for eggplant preparation.

# SWEET VEGETABLE MÉLANGE

2 large onions, sliced (about
   2 cups)
2 teaspoons olive oil
2 cups sliced carrot
2 small sweet potatoes, peeled
   and cubed (about 2 cups)

1½ tablespoons brown sugar
1 teaspoon cinnamon
¼ cup raisins
½ cup water

In a medium casserole, sauté onions in olive oil until soft.

Cover with carrots, then sweet potatoes.

Mix brown sugar, cinnamon, and raisins and sprinkle over vegetables.

Pour water over vegetables.

Cover and bake at 400°F for 45 minutes or until vegetables are tender.

*8 servings*
*Calories per serving: 85 total; 10 fat; 1 sat-fat*

# VEGETABLE SOUFFLÉ WITH TAHINI SAUCE

This recipe is a lot of work, but it's worth it. You may prepare the vegetable purée one or two days before serving and refrigerate it.

1 turnip, peeled and grated

6 carrots, peeled and grated

3 cups broccoli flowerets (about 1 head)

2 tablespoons margarine

2 tablespoons firmly packed brown sugar

1 tablespoon curry powder

½ teaspoon salt (optional)

¼ teaspoon freshly ground black pepper

⅛ teaspoon grated nutmeg

### Tahini Sauce

1 clove garlic

1 tablespoon parsley

3 tablespoons tahini (sesame seed paste)*

1 cup nonfat yogurt

1 tablespoon fresh lemon juice

½ tablespoon fresh dill or ½ teaspoon dried

4 egg whites

## The Vegetable Purée

Steam turnip and carrot 2–3 minutes or until tender. Set aside.

Steam broccoli flowerets about 5 minutes or until tender.

Purée turnip, carrot, and broccoli in food processor or blender until smooth. Set aside.

Melt margarine in a large skillet over low heat.

Stir in brown sugar until well blended.

Stir in curry powder, salt, pepper, and nutmeg.

Add puréed vegetables and mix well, stirring frequently until most moisture has evaporated.

Cool. (Cover and refrigerate if you wish to finish dish later.) While vegetable purée is cooling, make tahini sauce.

---

*Available at Mideastern food stores and many supermarkets.

### The Tahini Sauce

Chop garlic and parsley in food processor or blender.

Add tahini, yogurt, lemon juice, and dill.

Blend until smooth. Chill.

### The Soufflé

Preheat oven to 450°F. Grease a 1- or 2-quart casserole with margarine.

Beat egg whites until stiff but not dry.

Fold vegetable purée into egg whites, ⅓ at a time. Place in baking dish and bake at 450°F for 15 minutes.

Reduce heat to 350°F and bake for 30 minutes more or until puffed and golden brown.

Serve with tahini sauce.

*8 servings*

| *Calories per serving:* | *Total* | *Fat* | *Sat-fat* |
|---|---|---|---|
| | 75 | 22 | 5 |
| Tahini sauce per tablespoon | 20 | 11 | 1 |

# STEAMED VEGETABLES WITH DIJON-YOGURT SAUCE

The Dijon-Yogurt Sauce is so super-easy and delicious, you can eat it every day with any steamed vegetable.

Any vegetable, about ¾–1 cup
   per person

1 cup plain yogurt
2–4 teaspoons Dijon mustard

### Vegetable

Prepare vegetable for steaming by peeling and slicing if necessary or cutting off the stalk and cutting into bite-size flowerets, etc.

Place about 1 inch of water in a saucepan and turn heat to high. Insert metal steamer, spreading its "petals." Place cut-up vegetables on steamer.

Cover saucepan and heat water to boiling. Lower heat and steam vegetable until tender.

### Sauce

Mix 2 teaspoons mustard into yogurt and taste. If you want a stronger taste, add more mustard.

Spoon 1–2 tablespoons sauce over cooked vegetable. Refrigerate rest of sauce.

*1 cup sauce*
*Calories per tablespoon: 8 total; 0 fat; 0 sat-fat*

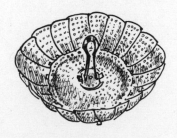

# ARTICHOKES

Artichokes make a great appetizer. Your family will gobble them up and then fight for the delectable hearts. Watch out for the margarine. It's 90–100 fat calories per tablespoon.

**1 artichoke for two people          Margarine**

Trim stem and pull off small leaves at base of artichoke.

With scissors, cut off tips of bottom leaves.

Drop artichoke into a large pot of boiling water and boil slowly for 40–45 minutes or until a leaf will pull off easily.

To eat an artichoke, pull off a leaf, dip it into a small bowl of melted margarine, and scrape the leaf between your teeth to extract the "meat." Discard the leaf.

When no more edible leaves are left, you have reached the heart. Remove excess leaves and scrape off hairy fibers above the heart. Dip heart in margarine or eat it plain.

| *Calories per serving:* | *Total* | *Fat* | *Sat-fat* |
|---|---|---|---|
| Artichoke | 26 | 0 | 0 |
| Margarine per tablespoon | 90 | 90 | 18 |

---

### Beans

If you have been avoiding beans because eating them produces more gas than you care to discuss, here is a way to prepare dried beans (except lentils and split peas) that reduces their gas-producing potential.

1. Rinse beans and pick out foreign matter.
2. Pour boiling water over beans and let them soak for four hours.
3. Drain beans and cook in fresh water.

---

## CURRIED BEANS

2 cups dried beans (½ cup each chickpeas, black-eyed peas, pinto beans, small red chili beans, or any combination)
1 teaspoon minced ginger root
1 cup chopped onion
1 teaspoon olive oil

1 cup chopped tomato
1 teaspoon coriander
2 teaspoons cumin
1 teaspoon turmeric
¼ teaspoon cayenne pepper
1 teaspoon salt (optional)
2 tablespoons tomato paste

Place dried beans in a large bowl or casserole. Rinse and remove any foreign matter.

Cover beans with boiling water and soak for at least 4 hours.

Drain water. Cover beans with fresh water and simmer for 40–60 minutes or until tender. Drain.

In a skillet, sauté ginger and onion in olive oil until soft.

Stir in tomato, coriander, cumin, turmeric, cayenne pepper, salt, and tomato paste.

Add beans and stir periodically for about 5 minutes. If beans become too dry, add a few tablespoons of water.

*11 half-cup servings*
*Calories per serving: 137 total; 7 fat; 1 sat-fat*

## SESAME BROCCOLI

| | |
|---|---|
| 1 tablespoon soy sauce | 2 heads broccoli, cut into |
| 1 tablespoon sesame oil | flowerets |
| ¼ cup dry sake or vermouth | 1 tablespoon sesame seeds, |
| 2 teaspoons honey | toasted |

Combine soy sauce, sesame oil, wine, and honey in a bowl. Set aside.

Steam broccoli until tender.

Toss broccoli and dressing together.

Sprinkle sesame seeds over broccoli and serve.

*8 servings*
*Calories per serving: 50 total; 20 fat; 3 sat-fat*

## CARAWAY CARROTS

Carrots are an excellent source of vitamin A. They keep well in the refrigerator and make great snacks. They are perfect for last-minute chefs because they cook quickly and taste wonderful with very little embellishment.

| | |
|---|---|
| 6 carrots, sliced (about 3 cups) | 2 teaspoons caraway seeds |
| 1 teaspoon olive oil | |

Place sliced carrots in a small saucepan with water to cover.

Gently simmer until carrots are soft. Drain.

Add margarine and mix until carrots are covered.

Stir in caraway seeds.

*6 servings*
*Calories per serving: 38 total; 7 fat; 1 sat-fat*

## CARROTS AND LEEKS

1 leek, cleaned thoroughly,                2 cups sliced carrots
    white bulb sliced                      ¼ teaspoon thyme
1 teaspoon olive oil

In a small saucepan, sauté leeks in olive oil. Add a splash of water and cook until tender.
Add carrots and thyme.
Cover and cook over low heat until carrots are tender.

*4 servings*
*Calories per serving: 51 total; 10 fat; 1 sat-fat*

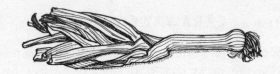

## CAULIFLOWER SAUTÉ

2 cups cauliflower flowerets                1 cup snow peas
2 cloves garlic, minced                     1 red pepper, sliced
1 small onion, sliced (about ¼             1 cup sliced mushrooms
    cup)                                    1 teaspoon oregano
1 teaspoon olive oil

Steam cauliflower until just tender. Set aside.
In large skillet or wok, sauté garlic and onion in olive oil until soft.
Add steamed cauliflower, snow peas, red pepper, mushrooms, and oregano and stir until heated through.

*6 servings*
*Calories per serving: 37 total; 7 fat; 1 sat-fat*

## CELERY AND MUSHROOMS

3 cups sliced celery                1 cup sliced onions
½ teaspoon salt (optional)          1 cup sliced mushrooms
2 teaspoons olive oil

Place celery and salt in a medium saucepan with water to cover.
Bring to a boil, reduce heat, and simmer for 8–10 minutes or until celery is tender.
Sauté onions in olive oil until golden.
Add mushrooms and stir for several minutes to blend flavors.
Drain celery and stir into onion-mushroom mixture.

*6 servings*
*Calories per serving: 27 total; 13 fat; 2 sat-fat*

## CHICKPEAS WITH LEMON AND HERBS

This dish also tastes good when made with black-eyed peas instead of chickpeas, and with parsley instead of oregano.

1 cup dried chickpeas               ½ teaspoon salt (optional)
¼ cup fresh lemon juice             1 teaspoon oregano
1 teaspoon olive oil                2 green onions, sliced

Place chickpeas in a large bowl or casserole. Rinse and remove any foreign matter.
Cover chickpeas with boiling water and soak for at least 4 hours.
Drain water. Cover chickpeas with fresh water and simmer for 40–60 minutes or until tender.
Combine lemon juice, olive oil, salt, oregano, and green onions and pour over chickpeas. Mix thoroughly.

*5 half-cup servings*
*Calories per serving: 154 total; 30 fat; 3 sat-fat*

### Cooking with Eggplant

Choose the blackest eggplant you can find. Peel it, cut it into bite-size pieces, and salt heavily. Place a heavy plate on top of the pieces to help squeeze out bitter juices. In 30–60 minutes, wash off the salt and gently squeeze eggplant pieces.

Steam eggplant in a vegetable steamer until tender. There are two advantages to steaming eggplant: it needs no oil (eggplant absorbs an enormous amount of oil) and thus saves hundreds of fat calories; and you can test the precooked eggplant for bitterness before using it in a recipe.

# KEEMA EGGPLANT

1 medium eggplant, cubed
   (about 4 cups)
1 cup sliced onion
1 teaspoon olive oil
2 teaspoons curry powder

3 tablespoons fresh lemon juice
1 tablespoon brown sugar
1 tablespoon ketchup
¼ cup water
1 cup canned chickpeas

Prepare eggplant according to directions above.

Sauté onion slices in olive oil until tender.

Stir in curry powder. Add eggplant.

Combine lemon juice, brown sugar, ketchup, and water and stir into eggplant mixture. Cook for 5 minutes.

Add chickpeas and cook for 2 minutes more.

*6 servings*
*Calories per serving: 86 total; 7 fat; 1 sat-fat*

# HOT AND GARLICKY EGGPLANT

1 medium eggplant (about 1
 pound)
5 small, dried black Chinese
 mushrooms*
1 tablespoon chili paste with
 garlic*
1 tablespoon vinegar
½ tablespoon soy sauce

½ tablespoon double black soy
 sauce*
2 tablespoons dry sherry
½ teaspoon sugar
1 large green pepper, chopped
1 teaspoon olive oil
½ cup water

Prepare eggplant according to directions on page 148.

Place mushrooms in a small bowl and cover with boiling water.

After about 15 minutes remove mushrooms. Squeeze out excess water and discard stems. Slice mushrooms. Set aside.

Combine chili paste with garlic, vinegar, soy sauce, double black soy sauce, sherry, and sugar and set aside.

In a large skillet, sauté green pepper and mushrooms in oil. Add a splash of water and cook vegetables until tender.

Stir in eggplant.

Mix in soy sauce mixture until vegetables are covered, then stir in water.

Simmer for about 5 minutes.

*8 half-cup servings*
*Calories per serving: 25 total; 5 fat; 1 sat-fat*

---

*Available at Asian food stores and some supermarkets.

## EGGPLANT WITH A GREEK INFLUENCE

| | |
|---|---|
| 1 large or 2 small eggplants | 12 pitted black olives |
| 2 teaspoons olive oil | 1 teaspoon capers |
| ¼ cup fresh lemon juice | ½ teaspoon oregano |

Prepare eggplant according to directions on page 148. Taste steamed eggplant. If not bitter, proceed.

In a saucepan, combine eggplant, olive oil, lemon juice, olives, capers, and oregano.

Cook over low heat for 10 minutes or until heated through.

*6 servings*
*Calories per serving: 44 total; 28 fat; 4 sat-fat*

## GREEN BEANS BASILICO

| | |
|---|---|
| 3 cups green beans, trimmed and cut in half | 2 teaspoons olive oil |
| 1 clove garlic, minced | 1 teaspoon basil |
| ½ cup chopped onion | ½ teaspoon oregano |
| ½ cup chopped green pepper | ½ teaspoon salt (optional) |

In a pot of boiling water, cook green beans 5–10 minutes until tender but still crisp and bright green. Drain and set aside.

In a large skillet, sauté garlic, onion, and green pepper in olive oil until soft.

Stir in basil, oregano, and salt.

Stir in green beans.

*6 servings*
*Calories per serving: 42 total; 13 fat; 2 sat-fat*

## LENTILS AND POTATOES

Lentils, a type of legume, are both delicious and nutritious. They are rich in vitamin C, folic acid, and many minerals, including iron and calcium. They are a good source of soluble fiber, which has been shown to lower blood cholesterol slightly.

Lentils and Potatoes may be served at room temperature on a bed of lettuce or warm as a side dish.

| | |
|---|---|
| 1 cup lentils | 2 cloves garlic, minced |
| 1 cup peeled and cubed potato (about 1 medium potato) | ⅓ cup chopped onion |
| ½ teaspoon salt (optional) | 2 teaspoons olive oil |

Wash lentils and place in a medium saucepan with potatoes, salt, and water to cover.

Bring to a boil. Reduce heat, cover, and simmer for about 20–25 minutes or until vegetables are tender.

Drain and set aside.

In a large skillet, sauté garlic and onion in olive oil.

Stir in cooked lentils and potatoes and serve or refrigerate.

*6 servings*
*Calories per serving: 145 total; 16 fat; 3 sat-fat*

## BRAISED MUSHROOMS ORIENTAL

These mushrooms make a tasty hors d'oeuvre or side dish.

| | |
|---|---|
| 1 pound mushrooms, sliced | 4 teaspoons soy sauce |
| 2 teaspoons olive oil | 1 cup water |
| 2 teaspoons sugar | 1 teaspoon sesame oil |

Sauté mushrooms in olive oil until tender.

Stir in sugar, soy sauce, and water.

Cover and simmer for 25 minutes or until water is absorbed.

Add sesame oil.

*6 servings as a side dish*
*Calories per serving: 50 total; 22 fat; 2 sat-fat*

## OKRA-TOMATO GUMBO

1 pound young okra (no more
   than 3 inches long)
1 tablespoon lemon juice
2 teaspoons olive oil
¼ cup flour
4 fresh tomatoes, coarsely
   chopped

1 cup chopped onion
½ teaspoon pepper
½ teaspoon basil
½ teaspoon thyme
½ teaspoon cayenne pepper

Wash okra and trim stem ends.

Bring a large saucepan of water to a boil. Add okra and lemon juice. Cover and cook until tender, about 5 minutes. Drain and set aside.

In a large skillet, combine oil and flour. Heat on high until flour becomes rust-colored (not burned!).

Mix in tomatoes, onions, and spices. Add ¼ cup water. Add okra. Stir until sauce is thickened.

*12 half-cup servings*
*Calories per serving: 45 total; 7 fat; 1 sat-fat*

| Potatoes |
|---|

Of all vegetables, potatoes are probably the most maligned. Many people consider them highly caloric and devoid of nutritional value. What injustice! Potatoes are filled with vitamins (particularly folic acid, niacin, and vitamin C), minerals, and protein. Eaten plain, they have no fat and are extremely filling and delicious.

## BAKED STUFFED POTATOES

This recipe is for 2 large baking potatoes or about 1⅓ pounds. For 4 potatoes, double ingredients; for 6, multiply by 3, and so on. You may use any type of potato.

2 large baking potatoes, about 11 ounces each

½ cup low-fat (1%) cottage cheese

½ egg white

1 tablespoon mustard

1 tablespoon chopped onion

Freshly ground black pepper to taste

Scrub potatoes thoroughly. Bake at 425°F for 1 hour or until soft inside.

Slice potatoes in half. Carefully scoop out the potato and place in mixing bowl. Set skins aside.

Add cottage cheese, egg white, mustard, and onion. Beat until well combined.

Fill potato skins with potato mixture and place on ungreased baking sheet in oven or toaster oven.

Bake at 375°F for 10 minutes or until lightly browned.

*4 potato halves*
*Calories per potato: 123 total; 3 fat; 1 sat-fat*

## BOUILLON POTATOES

4 medium potatoes, peeled and
   cut into ⅜-inch-thick slices
½ cup canned beef broth or beef
   stock, defatted
1 teaspoon vinegar
1 tablespoon minced carrot
1 small onion, quartered

2 cloves garlic, peeled
2 sprigs parsley
1 bay leaf
½ teaspoon thyme
3 sprigs parsley, chopped
1 teaspoon minced garlic

Line bottom of a large skillet with sliced potatoes.

Combine broth, vinegar, carrot, onion, whole garlic, parsley sprigs, bay leaf, and thyme, and pour over potatoes. Add water just to cover potatoes.

Bring to a boil and cook until liquid is completely evaporated (about 20 minutes). Check frequently, as final evaporation occurs suddenly.

Sprinkle with chopped parsley and minced garlic and serve.

*4 servings*
*Calories per serving: 106 total; 0 fat; 0 sat-fat*

# CURRIED WHIPPED POTATOES

You need not add butter or margarine to make delectable whipped potatoes. In this recipe, sautéed onions, mustard seed, and cumin make a special and exotic dish. Leave out the onions and you have plain but scrumptious whipped potatoes at 0 fat calories per serving.

4 potatoes (about 2 lbs)          ½ teaspoon cumin
¾ cup chopped onions              1–4 tablespoons skim milk
1 teaspoon olive oil              Salt and freshly ground black
½ teaspoon mustard seed             pepper to taste

Peel potatoes, slice thinly, and place in a medium saucepan with water to cover. Bring to a boil and cook until tender.

Meanwhile, sauté onions in olive oil. Lower heat to medium and stir in mustard seed and cumin. Cook a few moments until onions are soft.

Drain potatoes. Beat with an electric mixer. Add milk, one tablespoon at a time, until potatoes are fluffy.

Mix in onions and salt and pepper to taste.

*4 servings*
*Calories per serving: 168 total; 10 fat; 1 sat-fat*

## CURRIED POTATOES, CARROTS, AND PEAS

2 cloves garlic, minced
½ cup chopped onion
1 teaspoon olive oil
1 cup coarsely chopped
    tomato
1 teaspoon turmeric
½ teaspoon coriander
½ teaspoon cumin

¼ teaspoon cayenne pepper
    (optional)
½ cup water
2 cups sliced carrots
4 cups peeled and cubed baking
    potatoes
½ cup water
1 cup frozen peas

In a large saucepan or casserole, sauté garlic and onions in olive oil until soft.

Stir in tomato and spices. Add ½ cup water.

Mix in carrots and potatoes until well covered with sauce.

Add water and bring to a boil. Reduce, heat, cover, and simmer for about 10 minutes, stirring occasionally. Remove cover, add peas, and continue cooking until carrots and potatoes are tender.

*14 half-cup servings*
*Calories per serving: 31 total; 3 fat; 0 sat-fat*

# POTATOES LYONNAISE

2 pounds boiling or all-purpose
   potatoes (about 4 large)
½ tablespoon margarine
½ teaspoon salt (optional)
¼ teaspoon freshly ground black
   pepper

1½ cups sliced onion (about 2
   onions)
1 teaspoon olive oil
¼ cup chopped parsley

Peel and halve potatoes. Cut into ¼-inch-thick slices and steam or boil until just tender (about 10 minutes).

Melt margarine in a large skillet. Add potato slices and cook for 15 minutes, shaking pan periodically. After 10 minutes, add salt and pepper. Turn potatoes.

In a small skillet, sauté onions in olive oil until browned.

Add onions and parsley to potatoes and cook for 5 minutes more.

*8 servings*
*Calories per serving: 63 total; 11 fat; 2 sat-fat*

# POTATO SKINS

Leslie Goodman-Malamuth of the Center for Science in the Public Interest devised this recipe as a substitute for the fat-filled potato skins you often find in restaurants. Not only is this recipe quick and easy, the resulting potatoes are scrumptious.

4 large potatoes
1 teaspoon olive oil (optional)

Paprika to taste

Preheat oven to 450°F.

Scrub potatoes well, cut lengthwise into six wedges the size and shape of dill pickle spears, and dry on a paper towel.

In a large bowl, toss potato spears with olive oil until well covered.

Spread potatoes on a baking sheet, dust with paprika, and bake for 20–30 minutes or until fork-tender.

*6 servings (these are so good, 2 people can easily finish them off!)*
*Calories per serving: 66 total; 7 fat; 1 sat-fat*

---

### Sweet Potatoes

Sweet potatoes are often considered a fattening treat. They are a healthy treat, but not fattening. One sweet potato has no fat and is chock-full of vitamins A and C and many minerals.

---

## SWEET POTATOES WITH ORANGES, APPLES, AND SWEET WINE

4 cups sweet potatoes, peeled
  and cut into ½-inch slices
1 apple, peeled and diced
1 orange, peeled and cut into
  bite-size pieces

¼ cup brown sugar
1 cup sweet wine, sweet
  vermouth, or Chinese rice
  wine
10 whole cloves

Preheat oven to 375°F.

Place sweet potato slices in a saucepan with water to cover. Bring to a boil. Reduce heat, cover, and simmer until just tender when pierced with a fork.

Drain sweet potatoes. Reserve 1 cup liquid. Place sweet potatoes in a casserole with liquid.

Mix apple, orange, brown sugar, wine, and cloves.

Pour mixture over sweet potatoes.

Bake, covered, for 30 minutes or until apples are tender.

*6 servings*
*Calories per serving: 135 total; 0 fat; 0 sat-fat*

# SWEET POTATOES WITH MAPLE-BUTTERMILK DRESSING

For each person:

1 small sweet potato
1 teaspoon maple syrup

1 teaspoon nonfat buttermilk

Clean potato, prick with a fork, and bake for 60 minutes or until soft.

Mix maple syrup and buttermilk.

Split potato and mash the inside.

Mix in maple syrup mixture.

*Calories per sweet potato: 120 total; 0 fat; 0 sat-fat*

# SWEET POTATOES À L'ORANGE

Keep sweet potatoes on hand so you can whip up this wonderful, EASY recipe at the last moment. In the time it takes to boil the potatoes, you have created a healthy, delicious side dish.

2 pounds sweet potatoes
½ cup orange juice

1 orange (optional)

Peel and cut sweet potatoes into ½-inch slices. Place in saucepan with water to cover and boil until tender (about 20–30 minutes). Drain.

With an electric beater, begin beating sweet potatoes.

Slowly add orange juice and beat until creamy. Add more orange juice than you think you will need to make the potatoes fluffy, but do it slowly so you don't drown them.

Cut orange into pieces and mix by hand into whipped sweet potatoes.

*8 half-cup servings*
*Calories per serving: 125 total; 0 fat; 0 sat-fat*

## BRANDIED SWEET POTATOES

3 pounds sweet potatoes
⅔ cup brown sugar
¼ cup water

¼ cup raisins
⅓ cup brandy

Peel and cut sweet potatoes into ½-inch slices. Place in a medium saucepan, cover with water, and boil until just tender. Drain and place in a casserole.

Preheat oven to 350°F.

Mix sugar, water, and raisins together and bring to a boil.

Mix in brandy and pour over sweet potatoes.

Bake, uncovered, for 30 minutes.

Spoon syrup from bottom of casserole over potatoes.

*12 half-cup servings*
*Calories per serving: 175 total; 0 fat; 0 sat-fat*

## FLUFFY SWEET POTATOES

3 sweet potatoes (to make 2
   cups mashed)
⅔ cup orange juice
½ teaspoon grated orange rind

2 tablespoons brown sugar
1 tablespoon margarine, melted
1 egg yolk
2 egg whites

Peel sweet potatoes, cut into chunks, place in a medium saucepan, and cover with water.

Bring to a boil, then reduce heat and simmer until tender (about 10–15 minutes).

Preheat oven to 375°F. Grease a casserole with margarine.

Drain potatoes and mash in a large bowl.

Mix in juice, rind, sugar, melted margarine, and egg yolk.

Whip egg whites until stiff but not dry. Fold into sweet potato.

Pour sweet potato mixture into casserole and bake for 30 minutes.

*6 servings*
*Calories per serving: 118 total; 23 fat; 8 sat-fat*

## SPICED SWEET POTATOES

This recipe needs no fat to make it delicious.

| | |
|---|---|
| 2 pounds sweet potatoes | ¼–½ teaspoon cinnamon |
| 1 tablespoon brown sugar | ¼–½ teaspoon salt (optional) |
| ¼ teaspoon ground cloves | 6 tablespoons nonfat buttermilk |

Peel and thinly slice sweet potatoes. Place in saucepan, cover with water, and boil until tender (about 10–20 minutes).

Drain and place in the bowl of an electric mixer.

Add sugar, spices, salt, and 2 tablespoons of the buttermilk. Beat until fluffy.

Mix in remaining buttermilk.

*8 half-cup servings*
*Calories per serving: 135 total; 0 fat; 0 sat-fat*

## ROASTED RED PEPPERS

The intense, distinct taste of roasted red peppers adds flavor to many dishes. They are easy to prepare. You can use them in dishes like Jambalaya (page 64) or just marinate them in vinegar, basil, and a little olive oil.

Red peppers

Cut peppers in half, cut off stem, and remove seeds and membranes.

Turn on broiler.

Place pepper halves on wire rack, cut side down, about 6 inches from broiler coil. Broil until completely charred, about 10–15 minutes.

The blackened skin should peel off easily. If not, place peppers in a bowl with a plate on top for several minutes so that the steam can loosen the skin.

*Calories per pepper: 18 total; 0 fat; 0 sat-fat*

> ### Spinach
>
> Spinach is an excellent source of vitamin A. It is also rich in vitamin C and iron. It may be eaten raw in a salad or cooked in many interesting ways.

## SPINACH ORIENTAL

10 ounces fresh spinach, washed
  and shredded
1 teaspoon olive oil

1 teaspoon chopped ginger root
1 teaspoon double black soy
  sauce*

In a large skillet, lightly sauté spinach in oil until soft.
Stir in ginger and soy sauce.

*4 servings*
*Calories per serving: 30 total; 10 fat; 1 sat-fat*

## SPINACH AND TOMATOES

10 ounces fresh spinach, washed
  and shredded
2 cloves garlic, minced

1 teaspoon olive oil
1 tomato, diced
1 tablespoon raisins

In a medium saucepan, cook spinach in a cup of water until tender (about 2 minutes). Drain well and chop coarsely.
Sauté garlic in olive oil.
Mix in spinach.
Add tomatoes and raisins and heat through.

*4 servings*
*Calories per serving: 40 total; 9 fat; 1 sat-fat*

---

*Available at Asian food stores and some supermarkets.

---

### Squash

Squash, both winter and summer varieties, is rich in vitamin A, vitamin C, niacin, and iron. Squash is delicious when simply baked, boiled, or steamed and enhanced with a little margarine and freshly ground pepper. Or it may be prepared in a variety of other interesting ways.

---

## AFGHAN SQUASH

½ cup sliced onion
1 teaspoon olive oil
½ teaspoon salt
½ teaspoon cumin
½ teaspoon coriander

¼ teaspoon cardamom
¼ teaspoon ground cloves
1 butternut squash, peeled and
    cubed (about 3 cups)

Sauté onion in olive oil in a small casserole.
Stir in salt, cumin, coriander, cardamom, and cloves.
Add squash and 1 cup water.
Cook until tender (about 25 minutes).

*8 servings*
*Calories per serving: 25 total; 5 fat; 1 sat-fat*

## BUTTERNUT OR ACORN SQUASH

Don't be put off by the dull cream exterior of a butternut squash. Cut it in half and you will find a beautiful, deep orange interior. As a rule of thumb, one small squash (1–1½ pounds) serves two people.

| | |
|---|---|
| 1–2 small–medium butternut or acorn squash | 1 teaspoon margarine (optional) |
| 1 cup boiling water | Freshly ground black pepper to taste |

Preheat oven to 400°F.

Cut squash in half and scoop out seeds and fibers.

If you are cooking acorn squash, slice a small piece off the bottom of each half so that it will not roll over on the plate.

Place squash halves, cut-side down, in a shallow baking pan.

Pour boiling water into pan and cover tightly with aluminum foil.

Bake for 45 minutes or until squash is very soft when pierced with a fork. Keep squash covered with foil until ready to serve to retain moisture.

Before serving, place ½ teaspoon margarine on each half. (It is delicious without margarine.)

Grind pepper over squash and serve.

*2–4 servings*

| Calories per half squash: | Total | Fat | Sat-fat |
|---|---|---|---|
| | 40 | 0 | 0 |
| With margarine | 55 | 15 | 3 |

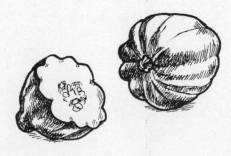

# SPAGHETTI SQUASH WITH TOMATO SAUCE

Spaghetti squash looks like an ordinary yellow squash — until you bake it. Inside, the pulp separates into long, thin strands like spaghetti. Use spaghetti squash as a healthy, vitamin-rich, delicious pasta. Top it with the tasty sauce below, Sweet Red Pepper Sauce (page 105), or Dijon-Yogurt Sauce (page 142).

1 spaghetti squash (about 3 lbs)

### Tomato Sauce

¼ cup sliced onion

1–2 teaspoons minced garlic

1 teaspoon olive oil

¼ cup chopped parsley

2 cups chopped cherry tomatoes
   (or regular tomatoes)

¼ teaspoon oregano

¼ teaspoon basil

¼ teaspoon cumin

¼–½ teaspoon red pepper flakes

¼–½ freshly ground black
   pepper

Salt to taste (optional)

### The Squash

Preheat oven to 350°F.

Cut squash in half lengthwise and scoop out seeds and fibers.

Place halves face down in shallow baking pan.

Bake for 45 minutes or until tender when poked with a fork.

### The Sauce

Meanwhile, in an 8-inch skillet, sauté onion and garlic in olive oil until soft. Lower heat to medium and stir in parsley.

Stir in tomatoes. Add oregano, basil, cumin, red pepper flakes, black pepper, and salt. Cook on medium heat, stirring occasionally, for about 10 minutes. Turn to low and let flavors blend for about 5–10 minutes. Set aside.

When squash is cooked, scrape inside with a fork to release spaghetti strands. Pile onto a plate (as you would spaghetti) and top with tomato sauce.

*4 servings*
*Calories per serving: 117 total; 10 fat; 2 sat-fat*

## CURRIED ZUCCHINI

You can use this basic recipe for any vegetable.

1 clove garlic, minced
½ cup chopped onion
1 teaspoon olive oil
½ teaspoon salt
½–1 teaspoon turmeric

¼–½ teaspoon cumin
½ teaspoon red pepper flakes
   (optional)
3 zucchini, sliced (about 3 cups)
2 tomatoes, chopped

In a large skillet, sauté garlic and onion in olive oil until soft.
Add salt, turmeric, cumin, and red peppers. Blend well.
Stir in zucchini and cook until tender.
Stir in tomatoes and serve.

*8 servings*
*Calories per serving: 23 total; 5 fat; 1 sat-fat*

## STEAMED ZUCCHINI MATCHSTICKS

2 small zucchini (or ½ small
   zucchini per person)
1 thick carrot, peeled

1 teaspoon margarine, melted
   (optional)
1 clove garlic (optional)

Cut zucchini and carrot into 2-inch lengths.
Place a zucchini section on a cutting surface, skin-side down.
Holding the sides of the section, slice lengthwise at ⅛-inch intervals. Hold slices together.
Roll the section one-quarter turn, making sure slices stay together.
Again, make parallel ⅛-inch slices lengthwise.
Result: zucchini matchsticks.
Repeat for remaining sections of zucchini and carrot.
Place zucchini sticks on top of carrot sticks in a vegetable steamer and steam until just tender (about 1 or 2 minutes).

*4 servings*

| Calories per serving: | Total | Fat | Sat-fat |
|---|---|---|---|
| | 17 | 0 | 0 |
| With margarine | 24 | 7 | 2 |

# ~6~
## Pizza, Quiche, and Chili

"OH, WOE IS ME," says the fat counter. "How can I go on without pizza and chili? Life will be bare." STOP! The following recipes for pizza, chili, quiche, and tortillas are delectable. And, except for the quiches, they will hardly graze your fat budget. So don't feel sorry for yourself. You *can* have your cake — or pizza — and eat it too!

# Pizza

You might think that a low-fat diet would eliminate pizza, but the following recipes will prove to you how fabulous low-fat pizzas can be. They make good snacks as well as main courses for lunch or dinner. Freeze leftovers (if there are any!). Then, in the future when you want a treat, heat the frozen slices in your toaster oven. We use low-fat (1%) cottage cheese. You may want to use nonfat mozzarella cheese instead.

To make pizza with a crisper crust, buy four inexpensive unglazed quarry tiles (each about a 5-inch square) at a tile store or purchase a pizza tile at a store that sells kitchen supplies. Pizza baked directly on hot tiles has a crunchier crust.

To slide the pizza onto the tiles, it helps to have a pizza peel, which looks like this:

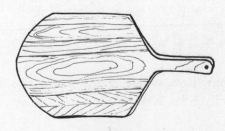

You may devise other gizmos to slide the pizza onto the tiles if you wish, but a pizza peel really works well. Of course, you may forgo both the tiles and the pizza peel and use a metal pizza pan or cookie sheet instead.

# PIZZA

### Dough

1 tablespoon active dry yeast
¼ cup warm water
Pinch of sugar
4 cups unbleached white flour

1 teaspoon salt (optional)
1 cup warm water
2 tablespoons olive oil

### Topping

2 cloves garlic, minced
Salt to taste
1½ cups tomato sauce
    (page 190)
2 cups sliced mushrooms
1½ sliced green peppers (about
    1½ cups)

1 cup sliced onion
1⅓ cups low-fat (1%) cottage
    cheese
3 teaspoons oregano

## The Dough

Place yeast, ¼ cup warm (but not hot) water, and sugar in a large bowl or the work bowl of your food processor. Let proof (become bubbly).

Mix in flour and salt.

Mix in 1 cup warm (but not hot) water and olive oil.

Knead or process until dough is smooth and elastic, adding more flour if needed.

Place dough in a large greased bowl, cover with a towel, and let rise for about 45 minutes.

While dough is rising, place tiles (see page 167) in oven and heat oven to 450°F.

After dough has risen, divide it into four parts, form each into a smooth ball, and cover for 10 minutes.

Roll dough into four small circles, 10 to 12 inches each. Wait 10 minutes more, then roll dough thinner.

### To Make Each Pizza

Cover pizza peel with a thin layer of cornmeal or grease pizza pan with oil.

Place one rolled circle of dough on pizza peel or in pizza pan.

Divide topping ingredients into four equal amounts.

Sprinkle garlic over surface of dough and sprinkle with salt.

Spoon tomato sauce over dough.

Arrange mushrooms, green peppers, and onions over tomato sauce.

Put cottage cheese on top (as if it were mozzarella).

Sprinkle with oregano.

Bake for 10–20 minutes or until crust is golden brown.

*4 pizzas, 4 slices per pizza*
*Calories per slice: 116 total; 4 fat; 1 sat-fat*

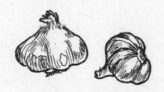

# CALZONE

A recipe that you can enjoy with no pangs of remorse. This seems like a lot of work, but once you do it, it goes quickly and is quite delicious. Bake a lot and freeze them. They taste best when you take them from the freezer and reheat them.

### Dough

| | |
|---|---|
| 1 tablespoon active dry yeast | 1–1½ teaspoons salt |
| Pinch of sugar | 1 cup skim milk |
| ½ cup warm water | 1 tablespoon olive oil |
| 3–4½ cups unbleached white flour | |

### Tomato Sauce*

| | |
|---|---|
| 1 teaspoon olive oil | 1 can (6 oz) tomato paste |
| 1 cup chopped onion | 2 teaspoons basil |
| 4 large cans (28 oz each) tomatoes | 1 teaspoon salt |

### Filling

| | |
|---|---|
| 1 clove garlic | 1 green pepper, sliced |
| Salt to taste | 1 cup sliced mushrooms |
| 1 cup low-fat (1%) cottage cheese | 1 cup sliced onion |

## The Dough

Place yeast, sugar, and warm water in food processor or large bowl and let proof.

Add 3 cups flour and salt and mix.

Add skim milk and olive oil and process until dough masses into a ball or knead until smooth and elastic. Add more flour if dough is too sticky.

---

*This recipe makes 8 cups of tomato sauce. You will need only about 1 cup for the calzone. Freeze the rest for future use in other recipes or as spaghetti sauce.

Place dough in a bowl greased with oil and cover with a towel. Let rise in a warm place for about 1 hour.

If you are using pizza tiles (see page 167), place them in preheated 450°F oven 30 minutes before baking pizza.

While dough is rising, make tomato sauce.

### The Tomato Sauce

Place olive oil in large saucepan.

Add onion and a splash of water and cook over low heat until tender.

Strain juice from canned tomatoes. (Freeze juice for soups.) Chop tomatoes (easily done in food processor).

Mix tomato paste into tomatoes. Add tomato mixture to saucepan.

Add basil and salt and cook until thick (about 45 minutes).

### To Make the Calzone

When dough has risen, divide it into 8 parts and form each part into a smooth ball. Cover with a towel or plastic wrap for about 10 minutes. It is important to let the dough "rest" or it will be difficult to roll flat.

Roll each ball into a flat circle. Wait 10 minutes more.

Roll each circle thinner. Place dough on floured surface or pizza peel sprinkled with cornmeal (see page 167).

Crush garlic and spread one-eighth over dough, then sprinkle with salt.

Spread about 2 tablespoons of tomato sauce over half the dough, leaving a border of ½ inch.

Spread 2 tablespoons cottage cheese evenly over tomato sauce.

Top with a few slices of green pepper, mushroom, and onion.

Fold top half of dough over and pinch top and bottom edges together.

Slide calzones onto hot tiles or cookie sheet.

Bake for about 10–20 minutes or until browned.

*8 calzoni*
*Calories per calzone: 296 total; 24 fat; 4 sat-fat*

# FOCACCIA

The whole-wheat flour in this pizza not only makes it healthier but also gives it a toasty taste and crunchy texture. Try it! It is easy and makes great snacks. Freeze it in snack-size slices.

### Dough

1½ teaspoons dry active yeast
½ teaspoon honey
1 cup warm water

2½ cups whole-wheat flour
¾ teaspoon salt (optional)
1 tablespoon olive oil

### Tomato Sauce

1 large can (28 oz) tomatoes, or
   3 large tomatoes
2 cloves garlic, minced
1 small onion, chopped
1 teaspoon olive oil

½ teaspoon oregano
¼ teaspoon basil
Ground hot cherry peppers
  (optional)

## The Dough

Place yeast, honey, and warm water in food processor or large bowl. Let proof.

Add flour, salt, and olive oil and process or knead until smooth and elastic, adding flour if needed.

Place dough in an oiled bowl, cover with a towel, and let rise in a warm place for about 1 hour.

Punch down dough and let it rest on floured counter for 10 minutes.

Grease a 10×15-inch cookie sheet with oil. Roll out dough (or press with your hands) onto the cookie sheet.

Pinch a rim around the edge. Cover with a towel and let rise for 30 minutes.

Meanwhile, make the tomato sauce.

## The Tomato Sauce

If using canned tomatoes, drain liquid and chop tomatoes. If using whole tomatoes, chop fine.

In a medium skillet, sauté garlic and onion in olive oil until tender.

Stir in tomatoes, oregano, and basil and let simmer until thick (about 10–15 minutes).

Let cool.

Preheat oven to 400°F.
Spread sauce over dough.
Add hot cherry peppers, if desired.
Bake for 20–25 minutes.

*12 pieces*
*Calories per piece: 113 total; 18 fat; 3 sat-fat*

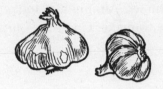

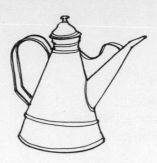

# PISSALADIÈRE

An onion pizza of Provence. Pissaladière makes a perfect luncheon dish, snack, or light dinner. Although it looks as if it takes a lot of work, it is quite simple to make. Cook the onions ahead to save time later.

### Filling

3 cups chopped onion
2 cloves garlic, minced

2 teaspoons olive oil

### Dough

1 teaspoon dry yeast
Pinch of sugar
¼ cup water
1–1½ cups unbleached white
   flour

½ teaspoon salt (optional)
¼ cup warm water
1 teaspoon olive oil

12 pitted black olives, halved

6 anchovies

## The Filling

In a small covered skillet, slowly cook onion and garlic in olive oil. Add a splash of water and cook until soft (about 30 minutes). Stir occasionally. Set aside. (You can refrigerate cooked onions for a few days.)

## The Dough

About 1¼ hours before serving, place yeast, sugar, and ¼ cup warm water in bowl or food processor. Let proof.

Mix in 1 cup of flour and salt.

Add ¼ cup warm water and olive oil and knead or process for 15 seconds.

Add more flour until dough is smooth and elastic.

Place dough in oiled bowl, cover with towel, and let rise for about 45 minutes.

After 35 minutes, preheat oven to 450°F.

On a greased round pizza pan or cookie sheet, roll out or push the dough into a 10-inch circle.

Spoon onions evenly over dough.

Starting from the center of the circle, place olive halves in lines like the spokes of a wheel.

Place anchovies between the lines of olives.

Bake for 20 minutes or until dough is slightly golden brown.

*8 slices*
*Calories per slice: 196 total; 29 fat; 5 sat-fat*

# Quiche

The word *quiche* conjures up images of dozens of eggs and tons of cream, ham, and cheese. The following wonderful much-lower-fat (but *not* low-fat) versions will surprise you. They make perfect appetizers or light meals.

## SPINACH QUICHE

Partially baked nonsweet quiche
   crust (page 276)
1 tablespoon chopped parsley
1 teaspoon basil
1 package (10 oz) fresh spinach
   (or frozen spinach, thawed)
1 cup low-fat (1%) cottage
   cheese
1 cup nonfat buttermilk

1 egg
1 egg white
1 tablespoon unbleached flour
½ teaspoon salt (optional)
¼ teaspoon freshly ground black
   pepper
¼ teaspoon grated nutmeg
2 tablespoons sliced green onion

Preheat oven to 375°F.

Combine parsley with basil (easily done in food processor) and set aside.

If using fresh spinach, wash leaves and tear off stems.

In a medium saucepan, cook fresh or thawed spinach for about 3 minutes in ½ cup boiling water. Drain. Squeeze all liquid out of spinach or quiche will be watery.

Combine cottage cheese, buttermilk, egg, egg white, flour, salt, pepper, and nutmeg in food processor or bowl.

If using processor, add spinach and process. If mixing in bowl, chop spinach finely and add to cottage cheese mixture.

Stir in green onion and parsley-basil mixture and pour into partially baked pie crust.

Bake for about 30 minutes.

*9 slices*
*Calories per slice: 177 total; 47 fat; 10 sat-fat*

# TOMATO QUICHE

Tomato Quiche is a winner. Elegant and unusual, it has an absolutely delicious Mediterranean flavor. If you are an anchovy-hater, do not avoid this recipe. The anchovies enhance the flavor but are not discernible.

Partially baked nonsweet quiche
crust (page 276)
⅓ cup chopped onion
1 teaspoon olive oil
1 large can (28 oz) + 1 small can
(16 oz) tomatoes
1 clove garlic, minced
¼ teaspoon basil
½ teaspoon oregano

½ teaspoon salt (optional)
6 sprigs parsley, stems removed
1 tin (2 oz) anchovies
1 egg
1 egg white
3 tablespoons tomato paste
12 large pitted black olives, cut
in half

In a medium skillet, sauté onion in olive oil until tender.

Meanwhile, drain juice from tomatoes. (Freeze the juice for future use.) Chop tomatoes and add to onion.

Mix in garlic, basil, oregano, and salt.

Increase heat to high. When tomato mixture begins to bubble, reduce heat to medium.

Cook tomatoes for about 50 minutes or until thick, stirring occasionally. You may have to reduce heat if mixture begins to boil. Make sure there is no excess liquid.

When sauce is very thick, remove skillet from heat. Cool sauce slightly.

Preheat oven to 375°F.

In a food processor or blender, mix parsley, anchovies, egg, egg white, and tomato paste.

Fold anchovy mixture into tomato sauce and pour into partially baked pie crust.

Artistically arrange olive halves on top of tomato mixture.

Bake quiche for 25–30 minutes or until puffy and browned on top.

*9 slices*
*Calories per slice: 183 total; 63 fat; 12 sat-fat*

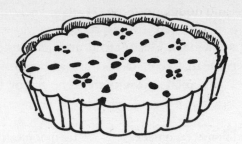

# TOMATO TART

Wonderful! So light and tasty.

### *Biscuit Crust*

1 cup unbleached white flour
1½ teaspoons baking powder
½ teaspoon salt (optional)

3 tablespoons olive oil
¼ cup nonfat skim milk

### *Tomato Filling*

1 pound fresh whole or cherry
  tomatoes or 1 large can
  tomatoes (28 oz)
¾ cup nonfat plain yogurt
1 small jar pimientos (2 oz),
  drained
2 teaspoons unbleached white
  flour

¾ teaspoon sugar
½ teaspoon salt
⅛–¼ teaspoon red pepper flakes
Freshly ground black pepper to
  taste
2 green onions, thinly sliced

## The Crust

Preheat oven to 425°F and lightly oil a 9-inch tart pan.*

Combine flour, baking powder, and salt in a mixing bowl or food processor bowl.

Add oil and milk and mix until a ball of soft dough forms.

Place dough on a floured piece of wax paper and roll into a ⅛-inch-thick circle, about 12 inches in diameter.

---

*A 9-inch tart pan with a removable bottom makes a very pretty crust that is easy to pop out. If you don't have a tart pan, a 9-inch pie plate will also work.

Flip the paper and dough onto the tart pan. Peel off wax paper and press dough into pan. If there is excess, roll it over the edge into a ridge.

Press a sheet of aluminum foil into dough to keep it from forming large bubbles during baking.

Bake 5 minutes and remove foil.

Bake 5–10 more minutes or until crust is evenly browned. Set aside.

## The Filling

Meanwhile, slice fresh tomatoes in half and squeeze out juices, or drain canned tomatoes and squeeze out juices.

Chop tomatoes into small pieces (preferably by hand — you don't want a purée). Set aside.

Combine yogurt, pimientos, flour, sugar, salt, red pepper flakes, and black pepper. Mix in green onions and tomatoes.

Spread tomato filling evenly over crust.

Put aluminum foil over edges of crust to prevent it from burning. Broil for about 4 minutes or until warmed.

*6 slices*
*Calories per slice: 173 total; 63 fat; 8 sat-fat*

# Chili

Chili is traditionally made with beef. You will not miss the beef in the following low-low-fat vegetarian recipes. They are delicious and filling — wonderful for a fall or winter day.

## PAWTUCKET CHILI

Ron eats this tasty chili with basmati rice every day for lunch. Nancy doubles the recipe so it lasts twice as long. Add the optional vegetables. They enhance the dish.

1 large can (40 oz) kidney beans
1 can (15 oz) chickpeas
2 cloves garlic, minced
1 medium onion, chopped
1 teaspoon olive oil
1 can (15 oz) tomato sauce
1–3 teaspoons oregano
½ teaspoon thyme
1 teaspoon cumin
½ teaspoon basil

1–2 tablespoons chili powder
1 large can (28 oz) whole
    tomatoes, chopped
1 green pepper, roughly chopped
    (optional)
2–4 cups torn spinach (optional)
1 can (14 oz) baby corns
    (optional)
1 tablespoon pickled jalapeño
    peppers (optional)

Drain kidney beans (reserve ½ cup liquid) and chickpeas. Rinse thoroughly to remove salt. Set aside.

Sauté garlic and onion in olive oil.

Mix in tomato sauce and spices.

Add tomatoes, beans, chickpeas, reserved liquid, and remaining ingredients and bring to a boil.

Simmer for about 20 minutes.

*8 one-cup servings*
*Calories per serving: 105 total; 9 fat; 1 sat-fat*

# CHILI NON CARNE

This is one of the best chili recipes we have ever tasted. It is filled with nutritious vegetables that provide texture but do not interfere with the delicious chili taste. Eat it in a bowl, mixed with chopped onions, tomatoes, and lettuce and sitting atop a bed of rice, or spoon it into pita bread with chopped onion, lettuce, and tomatoes.

Dried beans such as kidney beans and navy beans have been shown to have a modest effect in lowering blood cholesterol.

¾ cup chopped onion
2 cloves garlic, minced
1 teaspoon olive oil
2 tablespoons chili powder
¼ teaspoon basil
¼ teaspoon oregano
¼ teaspoon cumin
2 cups finely chopped zucchini
1 cup finely chopped carrot
1 large can (28 oz) tomatoes + 1
    small can (14½ oz) tomatoes,
    drained and chopped

1 can (15 oz) kidney beans,
    *undrained*
2 cans (15 oz each) kidney
    beans, *drained* and
    thoroughly rinsed
Chopped onions, tomatoes,
    lettuce, green peppers, for
    garnish

In a large pot, sauté onion and garlic in olive oil. Add a splash of water and cook until soft.

Mix in chili powder, basil, oregano, and cumin.

Stir in zucchini and carrots until well blended. Cook for about 1 minute over low heat, stirring occasionally.

Stir in chopped tomatoes and undrained and drained kidney beans.

Bring to a boil. Reduce heat and simmer for 30–45 minutes or until thick.

Top with chopped onions, tomatoes, lettuce, or green peppers.

*8 one-cup servings*
*Calories per serving: 117 total; 5 fat; 1 sat-fat*

# ~7~
# Pasta, Rice, and Other Grains

PASTA, BARLEY, RICE, and bulgur are filling and low in fat. As side dishes or complete meals, they add texture and variety to your eating.

## DAN-DAN NOODLES

½ pound fettuccine or linguine
1 teaspoon natural all-peanut peanut butter
2 teaspoons sesame oil
½ teaspoon minced garlic
½ teaspoon minced ginger root

½ teaspoon hot chili oil
2½ tablespoons white vinegar
1 teaspoon sugar
4 teaspoons soy sauce
2 green onions, chopped

Cook noodles according to package directions. Drain and refrigerate.

Combine peanut butter and sesame oil until mixture is completely smooth.

Mix in garlic, ginger, chili oil, vinegar, sugar, and soy sauce. Pour sauce over noodles. Sprinkle green onions over noodles and serve.

*4 servings*
*Calories per serving: 252 total; 32 fat; 5 sat-fat*

# ASPARAGUS PASTA

Asparagus Pasta makes a delightful luncheon dish, first course for an elegant meal, or light dinner. No one consuming this dish will believe how incredibly simple it is to make.

1 pound asparagus, sliced into
   1–2-inch pieces
3 tablespoons Dijon mustard
1 tablespoon olive oil
¼ cup thinly sliced shallots
1 clove garlic, minced
2 anchovy fillets

¼ teaspoon thyme
2 tablespoons chopped parsley
¾ pound very thin spaghetti or
   pasta of your choice
Salt and freshly ground black
   pepper to taste
1 cup sliced mushrooms

In a large pot of boiling water, cook asparagus until tender and still bright green (about 3 minutes).

Combine mustard, olive oil, shallots, garlic, anchovies, thyme, and parsley. Set aside.

Cook pasta. Drain, but reserve 1 cup of the cooking water.

Combine pasta with dressing. Add asparagus and mushrooms. Mix well. Add some of the cooking water if pasta is too dry. Add salt and pepper to taste.

Variation: Follow the original recipe but add two boneless, skinless chicken breasts that have been steamed and cut into bite-size pieces.

*4 servings*

| Calories per serving: | Total | Fat | Sat-fat |
|---|---|---|---|
| | 253 | 26 | 4 |
| With chicken | 296 | 30 | 5 |

# MANICOTTI

9 lasagna sheets or manicotti
   shells (lasagna sheets are
   easier to fill)
2 cups nonfat ricotta cheese
¼ cup Parmesan cheese

2 egg whites
2 tablespoons chopped parsley
½ teaspoon oregano
3 cups low-fat or nonfat tomato
   sauce*

Preheat oven to 350°F.

Cook pasta 8–10 minutes in boiling water, following directions on package. Drain and reserve in pot of cool water.

Combine ricotta, 3 tablespoons Parmesan cheese, egg whites, parsley, and oregano.

Drain pasta.

Spoon a thin layer of tomato sauce over the bottom of a 13×9×2-inch pan. Set aside.

If using lasagna, do the following with each sheet. First, cut sheet in half. In the center of one half, spoon in a heaping tablespoon of ricotta mixture. Fold the left third over ricotta. Fold the right third over. Place in pan, seam-side down, curly side toward long edges. Follow this procedure with second half of lasagna sheet. You will make 3 rows with 6 "manicotti" in each.

Spread remaining tomato sauce over pasta. Sprinkle with remaining Parmesan cheese.

Cover pan with foil and bake for 40 minutes. Remove foil and bake for 5 more minutes.

*18 manicotti*
*Calories per manicotti: 88 total; 7 fat; 0 sat-fat*

---

*Make half of the Basic Tomato Sauce recipe, page 190, or use commercial nonfat or low-fat tomato sauce. (Be sure to read labels. Many tomato sauces are high in fat.)

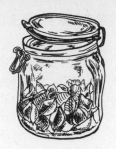

# PASTA MEXICALI

½ pound fancy pasta (fusilli,
   rigatoni, shells, etc.)
1 zucchini
½ cup chopped onion
1 teaspoon olive oil

1 teaspoon cumin
1 teaspoon chili powder
¼ teaspoon salt (optional)
1 red pepper, sliced
¼ cup tomato juice

Cook pasta according to package directions. Set aside.
Cut zucchini in quarters lengthwise. Slice into bite-size chunks.
Steam zucchini until just tender. Set aside.
In a small skillet, sauté onion in olive oil until soft.
Stir in cumin, chili powder, and salt.
Add onion mixture to pasta and mix well.
Add zucchini and red pepper. Add tomato juice and mix well.
Serve warm or at room temperature.

*6 servings*
*Calories per serving: 161 total; 7 fat; 1 sat-fat*

# PEASANT PASTA

Any combination of vegetables will do.

| | |
|---|---|
| 2 cups broccoli flowerets | 8 anchovy fillets |
| 1 cup cauliflower flowerets | 2 tablespoons olive oil |
| 1 zucchini, sliced | 1 large tomato, coarsely |
| 5 spears asparagus |   chopped |
| 20 green beans | 1 red pepper, coarsely chopped |
| ½ pound very thin spaghetti | 10–15 snow peas |
| ¼ cup chopped fresh parsley | 2 dried chili peppers or ½ |
| 2 cloves garlic |   teaspoon red pepper flakes |

Steam broccoli, cauliflower, and zucchini until tender and set aside.

Snap off bottoms of asparagus and boil for 1–2 minutes or until just tender. Set aside.

Submerge green beans in boiling water for 1–3 minutes or until just tender. Set aside.

While spaghetti is boiling (6 minutes), blend together parsley, garlic, anchovy fillets, and olive oil in a blender or food processor.

Drain spaghetti. Reserve 1 cup of water.

Stir anchovy sauce into spaghetti. If spaghetti is too dry, add a little water.

Stir in cooked vegetables, tomato, red pepper, and snow peas, until well covered with sauce.

Stir in red pepper flakes.

*6 servings*
*Calories per serving: 240 total; 41 fat; 6 sat-fat*

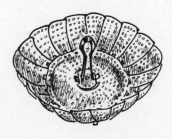

## PASTA WITH PESTO

Pesto hails from Genoa, Italy, where the salty soil makes the basil particularly wonderful. Even in the United States, pesto can be superb. It is easy to make and freezes well. If you don't have a food processor or blender, you can use a mortar and pestle.

| | |
|---|---|
| 2 cups fresh basil | 2 tablespoons Parmesan cheese |
| 3 cloves garlic | 1 tablespoon Romano cheese |
| 1 teaspoon salt | 1 package (16 oz) very thin |
| 2 tablespoons olive oil |    spaghetti |
| 1 tablespoon margarine | |

Prepare basil by rinsing it and tearing off the leaves. Discard the stems.

Chop garlic in a food processor or blender.

Add basil and salt. Process.

Add olive oil. Process until smooth. At this point you can put pesto aside for later use or freeze.

When ready to serve, mix margarine into pesto with a fork and blend well.

Blend in cheeses. Set aside.

Make spaghetti according to package directions.

Drain, but reserve 1 cup of the cooking water.

Mix pesto into pasta. If pesto is too dry, carefully stir in a small amount of spaghetti water.

*8 servings*
*Calories per serving: 287 total; 54 fat; 14 sat-fat*

## SALMON PASTA NIÇOISE

This delicious pasta may be eaten warm or cold. It is a meal in itself. (Beware: Although the dish is not high in sat-fat, it is high in total fat.)

3 large fresh tomatoes
1 egg or 1 egg white
1 tablespoon olive oil
4 tablespoons wine vinegar
1 tin anchovy fillets
1 large clove garlic, minced
6 large pitted black olives, halved

Salt to taste (optional)
Freshly ground black pepper to taste
8 ounces thin spaghetti
½ can (7½ oz) pink salmon*
1–2 slices red onion, coarsely chopped

Cut tomatoes into thick slices and quarter the slices.

Place egg in small pot, cover with water, and bring to boil. Let boil 1 minute or so. Cover pot, turn off heat, and let sit for 10 minutes until hard-boiled. Set aside or refrigerate. (You can do this step anytime during the day.)

Combine olive oil, vinegar, 4 smashed anchovy fillets, and garlic and pour over tomatoes. Mix in olives. Season with salt and pepper. Set aside to marinate for about 30 minutes or more.

Cook spaghetti, drain, and place in a large bowl. Stir tomato mixture into pasta. Break up salmon with a fork and add to pasta.

Slice egg (or remove egg yolk and slice white) and add along with onion and remaining anchovies.

*4 servings*

| Calories per serving: | Total | Fat | Sat-fat |
|---|---|---|---|
| With salmon | 325 | 70 | 13 |
| Using egg white | 320 | 57 | 9 |
| With tuna (6-oz can) | 340 | 62 | 9 |
| Using egg white | 325 | 50 | 6 |

---

*You may also substitute canned tuna in water for fewer total fat calories.

# PASTA WITH SPINACH-TOMATO SAUCE

One, two, three, and you have a delicious, healthy meal.

4 cloves garlic, pressed

1½ cups chopped onions

1 teaspoon olive oil

1 large can (28 oz) crushed
   tomatoes

1 tablespoon balsamic vinegar

½ teaspoon rosemary

¼ teaspoon cayenne pepper

¼ teaspoon basil

¼ teaspoon oregano

Freshly ground black pepper to
   taste

5 cups spinach, torn

1 tomato, cut into bite-size
   chunks

Pasta of your choice

In a large skillet, sauté garlic and onions in olive oil until soft. Add a splash of water to help cook them.

Stir in crushed tomatoes. Lower heat to medium.

Mix in balsamic vinegar, rosemary, cayenne, basil, oregano, and pepper.

Add spinach and stir until spinach is covered with sauce.

Add tomato.

Cook pasta according to package directions. Drain.

Pour sauce over pasta.

*6 cups*
*Calories per cup of sauce: 52 total; 7 fat; 1 sat-fat*

## SPAGHETTI SAUCE À LA SICILIA

Make a basic tomato sauce and add steamed eggplant and mushrooms for an appetizing spaghetti sauce that needs no ground meat.

1 small eggplant, peeled and cubed

6 cups Basic Tomato Sauce (below) or Zesty Fresh Tomato Sauce (page 192)

2 cups sliced mushrooms

12 ounces spaghetti

Prepare eggplant (see page 149) and steam until tender. Set aside.
In a medium saucepan, heat 6 cups of tomato sauce.
Stir in eggplant and mushrooms and cook 5 minutes more.
While sauce is cooking, prepare spaghetti according to package directions.
Pour tomato sauce over spaghetti and serve.

*6 servings*
*Calories per serving: 275 total; 10 fat; 1 sat-fat*

## BASIC TOMATO SAUCE

1 cup chopped onion
2 teaspoons olive oil
4 large cans (28 oz each) tomatoes, drained

1 can (6 oz) tomato paste
2 teaspoons basil
1 teaspoon salt (optional)

In a large saucepan, cook onion in olive oil until soft.
Chop tomatoes and add to onion.
Stir in tomato paste. (Tomatoes can easily be chopped and tomato paste blended in food processor.)
Stir in basil and salt.
Simmer until thick (about 45 minutes).
This tomato sauce freezes well.

*16 half-cup servings*
*Calories per serving: 32 total; 5 fat; 0 sat-fat*

# SPAGHETTI TOURAINE

1¼ pounds fresh tomatoes
4 cloves garlic, peeled
1 tablespoon + 1 teaspoon olive
  oil
Salt to taste
1 tablespoon minced carrot
1 tablespoon minced celery
1 tablespoon minced leek
1 tablespoon minced shallot
1 cup dry white wine or
  vermouth

Bouquet garni (2 parsley sprigs,
  ⅓ bay leaf, and ⅛ teaspoon
  thyme wrapped in
  cheesecloth)
½ cup + 2 tablespoons
  evaporated skim milk
¼ teaspoon salt (optional)
1 tablespoon dried tarragon (or
  fresh, if available)
10 ounces spaghetti

Place tomatoes in a large saucepan of boiling water. Immediately pour out hot water and pour in cold water.

Peel tomatoes, cut in half crosswise (not across the stem), squeeze out seeds and juice, and coarsely chop.

In a medium skillet, cook tomatoes and garlic in 1 tablespoon olive oil until reduced to a thick sauce (about 20 minutes). Stir occasionally. Add salt.

Meanwhile, heat 1 teaspoon olive oil in a small saucepan. Stir in carrot, celery, leek, and shallot.

Add wine and bouquet garni.

Cook until thick and stir in evaporated skim milk.

Remove bouquet garni and pour mixture through a sieve to strain out vegetables. Add tarragon.

Mix with tomato sauce and pour over pasta.

*4 servings*
*Calories per serving: 165 total; 40 fat; 5 sat-fat*

## ZESTY FRESH TOMATO SAUCE

Fresh tomatoes make this sauce special. It's fragrant, tasty, and simple to make.

1 medium onion, sliced
2–3 cloves garlic, minced
1 teaspoon olive oil
½ cup chopped parsley
4 cups chopped cherry tomatoes
   (or regular tomatoes)
½ teaspoon oregano

½ teaspoon basil
½ teaspoon cumin
½–1 teaspoon red pepper flakes
¼–½ freshly ground black
   pepper
Salt to taste (optional)

In a large skillet, sauté onion and garlic in olive oil until soft. Lower heat to medium and stir in parsley.

Stir in tomatoes. Add oregano, basil, cumin, red pepper flakes, black pepper, and salt. Cook at medium heat, stirring occasionally, for about 10 minutes. Turn to low and let flavors blend for about 5–10 more minutes.

*5 half-cup servings (approximately)*
*Calories per serving: 48 total; 8 fat; 1 sat-fat*

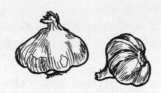

# FRIED RICE

2 egg whites
½ egg yolk
1 teaspoon + 1 teaspoon olive
    oil
3 green onions, cut into ¼-inch
    pieces

3 cups boiled rice (cold)
1 tablespoon soy sauce
¼ teaspoon sugar
¼ cup cooked diced chicken,
    shrimp, turkey, or
    combination

Beat egg whites and yolk together.

In a small skillet, scramble eggs in 1 teaspoon of olive oil. Set aside.

In a large skillet, sauté green onions in the remaining teaspoon of oil.

Add rice and mix thoroughly.

Stir in soy sauce, sugar, eggs, and meat.

*6 half-cup servings*
*Calories per serving: 154 total; 20 fat; 4 sat-fat*

# INDIAN RICE

1 teaspoon olive oil
2 cloves garlic, minced
1 tablespoon minced ginger root
¾ cup chopped onion
¼ teaspoon cardamom
¼ teaspoon caraway seeds

1 teaspoon coriander
¼ teaspoon cinnamon
¼ teaspoon ground cloves
¼ teaspoon salt (optional)
1½ cups long-grain rice
3¾ cup water

In a medium saucepan, heat olive oil.

Add garlic, ginger, onion, and a splash of water and cook until soft.

Mix in cardamom, caraway seeds, coriander, cinnamon, cloves, salt, and rice and blend well.

Add water, cover, and bring to a boil. Reduce heat and cook until all water is absorbed (about 25 minutes).

*12 half-cup servings*
*Calories per serving: 91 total; 5 fat; 1 sat-fat*

# RICE AND BEANS

A tasty combination that couldn't be healthier.

### Beans

2 cups dry pinto beans
⅔ cup chopped onion
2 bay leaves
8 cups cold water

1 teaspoon olive oil
4 cloves garlic, minced
½ teaspoon salt (optional)

### Rice

2 cloves garlic
½ cup chopped onion
2 medium tomatoes
2 cups long-grain rice
¼–½ teaspoon cayenne pepper
(optional)
Freshly ground black pepper to
taste

1 can (4 oz) diced green chili
peppers
2 cans (10¾ oz each) chicken
broth, defatted
1 cup water

### Garnish

¼ cup chopped cilantro

1 medium tomato, chopped

## Cook Beans

Discard stones and any other debris from beans. Wash beans, cover with water, and soak overnight.

Drain beans and put in a large pot with onion, bay leaves, and water.

Bring to a boil, cover, lower heat, and simmer for 1–2 hours or until very tender. Check periodically to see if you need to add more water.

## Prepare Rice

Chop garlic, onion, and tomatoes in a blender or food processor.

Combine with rice and spices in a medium saucepan. Turn heat to high.

Stir in chicken broth and water and bring to a boil. Turn heat to low and cover pot. Cook for about 20 minutes. Don't let rice get too dry.

When rice is cooked, stir in chilies.

### Prepare Bean Dish

Drain liquid from beans and reserve liquid. Set beans aside.

In a large skillet, heat oil. Add garlic and cook until you smell its wonderful aroma — about 1 minute.

Add 1 cup of beans and mash completely with the back of a spoon.

Stir in ½ cup of reserved liquid. Add remaining beans, mashing about half.

Stir in more liquid until desired consistency is reached. Heat for about 5 minutes, adding more liquid if necessary. Keep remaining liquid in case beans become too dry.

Serve heaping ½ cup of beans over 1 cup of rice.

Top with cilantro and tomato.

*8 servings (heaping half cup beans, one cup rice)*

| Calories per serving: | Total | Fat | Sat-fat |
|---|---|---|---|
| Beans | 175 | 10 | 1 |
| Rice | 190 | 1 | 0 |

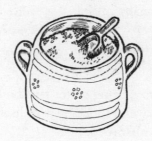

# LEMON RICE WITH SPINACH AND RED PEPPER

⅓ cup chopped onion
1 teaspoon olive oil
1 cup long-grain rice
½ teaspoon salt (optional)
2½ cups water

1 cup chopped spinach
2 tablespoons fresh lemon juice
1 red pepper, chopped (about ½ cup)

In a medium saucepan, sauté onion in olive oil until soft.

Mix in rice and salt. Add water and bring to a boil. Reduce heat to low or off and cover saucepan.

After 15 minutes, stir spinach and lemon juice into rice.

Cook for 10 minutes more or until liquid is completely absorbed.

Mix in red pepper and serve.

*8 half-cup servings*
*Calories per serving: 90 total; 5 fat; 0 sat-fat*

# OLIVE-ARTICHOKE RICE

3¾ cups water
1½ cups long-grain rice
½ teaspoon salt (optional)
1 tablespoon olive oil
1 tin (2 oz) anchovies (omit if you hate anchovies)

1 red pepper, sliced
½ cup artichoke hearts, diced
12 pitted black olives, sliced

In a medium saucepan, bring water to a boil.

Add rice and salt, cover, reduce heat to low, and cook for 25 minutes or until all water is absorbed.

Mix in remaining ingredients and cool to lukewarm.

*14 half-cup servings*
*Calories per serving: 88 total; 16 fat; 3 sat-fat*

# RICE PILAU WITH APRICOTS AND RAISINS

3 tablespoons slivered almonds
1 teaspoon olive oil
1 teaspoon minced ginger root
1 clove garlic, minced
¼ cup chopped onion
1 teaspoon salt (optional)
2 whole cloves

½ cinnamon stick
1 teaspoon turmeric
1½ cups long-grain rice
3¾ cups water
¼ cup apricots, sliced
2 tablespoons raisins

In a medium casserole, sauté slivered almonds in olive oil over medium heat until golden.

Add ginger, garlic, and onion and sauté until soft.

Mix in salt, cloves, cinnamon stick, and turmeric.

Add rice and stir until well coated.

Add water and bring to a boil. Cover, reduce heat to low (or off), and cook until water is absorbed (about 25 minutes).

Mix in apricots and raisins.

*14 half-cup servings*
*Calories per serving: 96 total; 11 fat; 1 sat-fat*

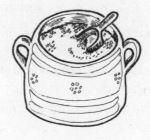

## BARLEY PLUS

An interesting alternative to rice.

¾ cup chopped onion
½ cup chopped mushrooms
2 teaspoons olive oil
1 cup pearl barley, rinsed

1 can (10¾ oz) chicken broth, defatted
½ teaspoon salt (optional)

Sauté onion and mushrooms in olive oil until tender. Stir in barley.

Add 1 cup of the chicken broth plus salt and bring to a boil. Cover and simmer for 25 minutes.

Add remaining broth plus water to equal 1 cup. Cook 25 more minutes until liquid is absorbed.

Fluff barley with a fork before serving.

*6 servings*
*Calories per serving: 150 total; 13 fat; 3 sat-fat*

## BULGUR WITH TOMATOES AND OLIVES

1 cup bulgur (cracked wheat)
2 teaspoons olive oil
1 cup tomato juice
1 cup water

1 tomato, chopped
¼ cup sliced green olives
2 stalks celery, chopped
3 green onions, sliced

In a large skillet, sauté bulgur in olive oil until bulgur begins to color and crackle.

Add tomato juice, water, and tomato and simmer until most liquid is absorbed (about 35 minutes).

Add olives, celery, and green onions and mix until heated through.

*9 half-cup servings*
*Calories per serving: 68 total; 12 fat; 1 sat-fat*

# ~ 8 ~
# Salads and Salad Dressings

## Salads

**SALADS ARE REFRESHING.** They can be nutritious and add texture to a meal. Salads by themselves generally contain very little fat. But beware of high-fat salad dressings! These culprits turn many a healthy salad into a fat-calorie extravaganza.

Gourmet food shops and supermarket deli-bars specialize in a variety of high-fat salads — pasta, rice, chicken, turkey, and fish salads. Here are a few salads you can make yourself and eat without hesitation.

### CUCUMBER SALAD

2 cucumbers, peeled and sliced thin
1 medium onion, sliced thin
½ teaspoon salt (optional)

1 teaspoon sugar
1 teaspoon fresh dill
1 cup white vinegar

Mix cucumbers and onion together in a ceramic or glass bowl.

Add salt, sugar, and dill to vinegar and pour over cucumbers and onion.

Chill 1 hour.

*6 servings*
*Calories per serving: 20 total; 0 fat; 0 sat-fat*

# BLACK BEAN AND CORN SALAD

4 cups frozen corn
2 cans (15 oz each) black beans
   or other beans
1 cup chopped red and/or green
   pepper
¼ cup pickled jalapeño pepper
   (optional)

½ cup white vinegar
½ teaspoon salt (optional)
½–1 teaspoon freshly ground
   black pepper
½–1 teaspoon chili powder

Cook corn until tender according to package directions.
Drain and rinse beans and place in bowl or casserole.
Mix in peppers.
Drain cooked corn and add to bean mixture.
Combine vinegar, salt, and spices and pour over corn and beans.
Mix well. Cover and refrigerate several hours.

*12 half-cup servings*
*Calories per cup: 102 total; 10 fat; 2 sat-fat*

# RED POTATO SALAD

4–5 red potatoes
½ cup nonfat yogurt
3 tablespoons low-fat
  mayonnaise

1 teaspoon tarragon
1 tablespoon white vinegar
1 teaspoon Dijon mustard
½ teaspoon salt (optional)

Scrub potatoes thoroughly. Steam until tender.
Meanwhile, combine remaining ingredients. Set aside.
Cut potatoes into chunks (do not remove skin).
Pour sauce over potatoes so they are thoroughly coated.
Serve warm or cold.

*6 servings*
*Calories per serving: 95 total; 5 fat; 0 sat-fat*

## CORIANDER CHICKEN SALAD

6 boneless, skinless chicken
   breasts
½ cup unbleached white flour
½ teaspoon salt (optional)
¼ teaspoon freshly ground black
   pepper

¼ teaspoon coriander
2 cups broccoli flowerets
2 tablespoons low-fat
   mayonnaise
2 tablespoons nonfat yogurt
2 teaspoons Dijon mustard

Shake chicken with flour, salt, and pepper and cook as in Tarragon-Raisin Chicken Salad (page 204).

Cut chicken into large chunks, mix with coriander, and set aside.

Steam broccoli until just tender.

Combine mayonnaise, yogurt, and mustard.

Mix dressing with chicken.

Stir in broccoli until coated with dressing.

*8 servings*
*Calories per serving: 110 total; 12 fat; 3 sat-fat*

## CHICKEN SALAD WITH SHALLOTS AND MUSHROOMS

3 boneless, skinless chicken
   breasts
¼ cup unbleached white flour
½ teaspoon salt (optional)
¼ teaspoon freshly ground black
   pepper

1 teaspoon olive oil
2 tablespoons white vinegar
2 teaspoons minced shallot
1 cup sliced mushrooms
1 teaspoon thyme
¼ teaspoon salt (optional)

Shake chicken with flour, salt, and pepper and cook as in Tarragon-Raisin Chicken Salad (page 204).

When chicken is cool enough to handle, cut it into bite-size pieces.

Combine remaining ingredients and pour over chicken.

Mix until chicken is well coated.

*4 servings*
*Calories per serving: 113 total; 20 fat; 4 sat-fat*

# DIJON CHICKEN-RICE SALAD

3¾ cups water
1½ cups long-grain rice
½ teaspoon salt (optional)
3 tablespoons Dijon mustard
3 tablespoons white vinegar
1 tablespoon olive oil

1½–2 cups diced green and/or
   red pepper
¼ cup pitted black olives, sliced
¼ cup sliced green onion
3 cooked chicken breasts, diced

In a medium saucepan, bring water to a boil.

Add rice and salt, reduce heat, cover, and simmer for 20–25 minutes or until water is absorbed.

Place rice in a bowl.

Combine mustard, vinegar, and olive oil and mix into rice.

Add green pepper, olives, green onion, and chicken and mix well.

This salad tastes best when tepid. If too dry, mix in a little water, 1 tablespoon at a time.

*6 one-and-a-half-cup servings*
*Calories per serving: 267 total; 34 fat; 7 sat-fat*

# ORIENTAL CHICKEN SALAD

4 boneless, skinless chicken
   breasts
¼ cup unbleached white flour
½ teaspoon salt (optional)
¼ teaspoon freshly ground black
   pepper
1 head broccoli, cut into
   flowerets (about 3 cups)

1 teaspoon walnut oil
3 tablespoons soy sauce
2 tablespoons dry vermouth
2 teaspoons minced ginger root
2 teaspoons chopped walnuts
2 cups mushrooms, sliced
1 head red-leaf or Boston lettuce

Shake chicken with flour, salt, and pepper and cook as in Tarragon-Raisin Chicken Salad (page 204).

When chicken is cool enough to handle, cut it into bite-size pieces. Set aside.

Steam broccoli flowerets until *just* tender.

Combine walnut oil, soy sauce, vermouth, and ginger in a large bowl.

Add walnuts, mushrooms, and chicken and mix until all are coated with sauce. Stir in broccoli.

Place some lettuce on each salad plate. Top with chicken salad.

*6 servings*
*Calories per serving: 140 total; 29 fat; 6 sat-fat*

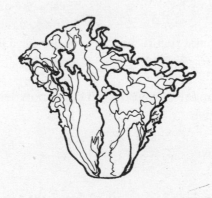

## TARRAGON-RAISIN CHICKEN SALAD

4 boneless, skinless chicken
  breasts
¼ cup unbleached white flour
½ teaspoon salt (optional)
¼ teaspoon freshly ground black
  pepper

2 tablespoons low-fat
  mayonnaise
2 tablespoons nonfat yogurt
2 teaspoons tarragon
2 tablespoons golden raisins

Preheat oven to 375°F.

Shake chicken in a plastic bag with flour, salt, and pepper to coat. Place chicken in a single layer in a shallow pan and bake until fully cooked, about 20–30 minutes.

When chicken is cool enough to handle, cut it into large chunks and set aside.

Combine mayonnaise, yogurt, tarragon, and raisins.

Add to chicken and mix until chicken is well coated.

*4 servings*
*Calories per serving: 146 total; 13 fat; 4 sat-fat*

## CURRIED TUNA SALAD WITH PEARS

1½ tablespoons low-fat
  mayonnaise
2 tablespoons nonfat yogurt
¼–½ teaspoon curry powder

2 cans (6½ oz each) water-
  packed tuna, drained
¼ cup diced pear
Lettuce

Combine mayonnaise, yogurt, and curry powder.

Mix into tuna fish.

Stir in pear.

Serve over lettuce.

*3 servings*
*Calories per serving: 154 total; 22 fat; 3 sat-fat*

# EASTERN SPINACH SALAD

1 package (10 oz) fresh spinach,
    washed and shredded
10 water chestnuts, sliced
3 green onions, sliced
1 cup sliced mushrooms
1 cucumber, peeled and sliced
    thin

1 tablespoon olive oil
2 tablespoons soy sauce
3 tablespoons fresh lemon juice
1½ tablespoons honey
1 tablespoon sesame seeds,
    toasted

In a salad bowl, combine spinach, water chestnuts, green onions, mushrooms, and cucumber slices.

Mix together olive oil, soy sauce, lemon juice, and honey and pour over salad.

Sprinkle with sesame seeds.

*8 servings*
*Calories per serving: 55 total; 20 fat; 3 sat-fat*

# TABBOULI

1 cup bulgur (cracked wheat)
3 cups boiling water
1 can (15 oz) chickpeas, drained
¼ cup fresh mint, minced, or 1
    teaspoon dried mint
2 teaspoons oregano
½ teaspoon salt (optional)
¼ teaspoon freshly ground black
    pepper

2 cloves garlic, minced
1 small onion, chopped
1 green pepper, chopped
2 medium tomatoes, chopped
1 tablespoon olive oil
3 tablespoons fresh lemon
    juice
¼ cup chopped parsley

Place bulgur in a large bowl and cover with boiling water.

Let stand for about 1 hour or until fluffy. Squeeze out excess water.

Add remaining ingredients to bulgur. Chill for at least 1 hour.

*14 half-cup servings*
*Calories per serving: 87 total; 10 fat; 2 sat-fat*

# SALADE NIÇOISE

Salade Niçoise is a meal in itself. Ours is a lower-fat version of those served on the Riviera.

### Dressing

1 clove garlic, minced
1 tablespoon lemon juice
1 tablespoon white vinegar
½ tablespoon Dijon mustard

½ teaspoon basil
¼ teaspoon salt (optional)
1½ tablespoons olive oil

### Salad

2 potatoes
1½ cups green beans, tips
  removed and cut in half
1 small head red-leaf or Boston
  lettuce, shredded
2 tomatoes, cut into eighths

Whites from 2 hard-boiled eggs
2 tablespoons pitted black olives
1 tablespoon capers
1 oz anchovy fillets
3 oz water-packed solid white
  tuna, drained

Combine all dressing ingredients in a jar and shake vigorously. Set aside.

Steam potatoes until tender, peel, and cut into bite-size pieces.

Mix potatoes with 1 teaspoon dressing and set aside.

Cook green beans in boiling water for 5 minutes or until just tender and bright green.

Put lettuce and tomatoes in a large salad bowl and toss with the remaining dressing.

Add potatoes, green beans, egg whites, olives, capers, anchovies, and drained tuna and mix until well coated with dressing. Traditionally each vegetable is segregated on the plate. We prefer them mixed into the salad.

*5 servings*
*Calories per serving: 128 total; 43 fat; 6 sat-fat*

# SHRIMP AND MACARONI SALAD

### Green Goddess Dressing

1 teaspoon tarragon leaves

1 tablespoon tarragon vinegar or
  white vinegar

1 tablespoon lemon juice

1 green onion

3 tablespoons parsley

2 teaspoons anchovy paste or
  anchovy fillets

2 teaspoons sugar

½ teaspoon salt (optional)

1 cup nonfat yogurt

### Salad

½ pound shrimp

1½ cups uncooked macaroni

1 tomato

1 stalk celery

Place tarragon, vinegar, and lemon juice in a blender.

Wait 5 minutes, then add green onion, parsley, anchovies, sugar, salt, and yogurt. Blend until smooth.

Refrigerate dressing while you prepare the rest of the ingredients.

Peel and devein shrimp. Place in a small pot of boiling water and boil for a few minutes until they change color and are cooked through. Refrigerate.

Prepare macaroni as directed on the package.

While macaroni is cooking, cut tomato into bite-size pieces. Set aside.

Dice celery. Set aside.

Drain macaroni and place in a medium casserole or bowl. Cool for a few minutes. Add shrimp, tomatoes, and celery.

Mix in Green Goddess Dressing until all salad ingredients are covered.

### Salad

*6 one-cup servings*
*Calories per serving: 124 total; 8 fat; 1 sat-fat*

### Dressing

*1¼ cups*
*Calories per tablespoon: 8 total; 0 fat; 0 sat-fat*

# INDONESIAN VEGETABLE SALAD

2 cups shredded lettuce or
  Chinese celery cabbage
1 cup sliced carrot
1 cup green beans, cooked

in boiling water until just
  tender
2 tomatoes, sliced
1 cucumber, peeled and sliced

### Dressing

1 tablespoon sliced green onion
½ tablespoon olive oil
4 tablespoons natural all-peanut
  peanut butter
1 clove garlic, minced
½ teaspoon red pepper flakes

1 bay leaf
1 slice lemon
1 teaspoon sugar
½ teaspoon salt
¾ cup skim milk
2 tablespoons water

Place lettuce on a platter.

Artistically arrange carrots, green beans, tomatoes, and cucumber over lettuce. Cover with plastic wrap and chill in refrigerator.

In a small saucepan, sauté green onion in olive oil.

Mix in peanut butter, garlic, red pepper flakes, bay leaf, lemon, sugar, and salt until peanut butter starts to melt.

Gradually blend in skim milk. Cook over low heat, stirring constantly, until thick. Remove bay leaf and lemon. Chill dressing.

Before serving, dilute dressing with water, if necessary.

Pass platter and dressing separately so each person can take what he or she wants.

### Salad

*6 servings*
*Calories per serving: 32 total; 0 fat; 0 sat-fat*

### Dressing

*¾ cup*
*Calories per tablespoon: 43 total; 30 fat; 5 sat-fat*

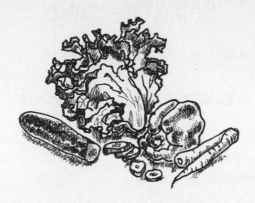

## SPECIAL VEGETABLE SALAD

Chock full of colorful vegetables, this refreshing, tasty salad is a pleasure to look at as well as to eat.

1 large cucumber, cubed (2 cups)

2–3 carrots thinly sliced (¾ cup)

¾ cup red pepper, roasted* or plain, coarsely chopped

¾ cup coarsely chopped red onion

1 can (15½ oz) chickpeas, drained and rinsed

1 tomato, coarsely chopped

½ cup Tangy Salad Dressing (see page 210)

Freshly ground pepper to taste

Salt to taste (optional)

Combine all ingredients and mix so that vegetables are well covered. Refrigerate and chill or serve right away.

*6 one-cup servings*
*Calories per cup: 105 total; 12 fat; 3 sat-fat*

*See Roasted Red Peppers, page 161.

# Salad Dressings

Who says fat-free dressings can't be delicious? Here's proof.

## TANGY SALAD DRESSING

¾ cup balsamic vinegar
¼ cup Dijon mustard
1–2 tablespoons honey

1 teaspoon lemon juice
5 garlic cloves, minced or
   pressed

Put all ingredients into a jar that has a cover. Cover and shake vigorously until well combined.

*1 cup dressing*
*Calories per cup: 194 total; 0 fat; 0 sat-fat*
*Calories per tablespoon: 12 total; 0 fat; 0 sat-fat*

## CREAMY SALAD DRESSING

¼ cup balsamic vinegar
½ cup nonfat yogurt
¼ cup Dijon mustard
1–2 tablespoons honey

1 teaspoon lemon juice
5 garlic cloves, minced or
   pressed

Put all ingredients into a jar that has a cover. Cover and shake vigorously until well combined.

*15 tablespoons dressing (approximately)*
*Calories per 15 tablespoons: 209 total; 0 fat; 0 sat-fat*
*Calories per tablespoon: 14 total; 0 fat; 0 sat-fat*

# ~9~
# Dips, Sandwiches, and a Drink

SOUR CREAM NEED NOT BE the basis for your dips and sandwich spreads. Sour cream has 434 fat calories per cup. In its place, use non-fat or low-fat yogurt or cottage cheese, eggplant, or chickpeas for delicious low-fat and nonfat dips and spreads.

## CREAMY GINGER-CURRY DIP

A good substitute for sour cream or cream cheese is yogurt cheese (page 213). Made with nonfat yogurt, it adds 0 fat to your dish. Remember: In this recipe, allow 12–24 hours to make the yogurt cheese.

| | |
|---|---|
| 2 cups nonfat yogurt | 2 tablespoons cider vinegar |
| ⅓ cup orange marmalade | ¼ teaspoon salt (optional) |
| 2 teaspoons brown sugar | ¼ teaspoon curry powder |
| 1½ teaspoons granulated sugar | ¼ teaspoon powdered sugar |

Make yogurt cheese (page 213). Let yogurt drain in the refrigerator for about 12–24 hours.

When yogurt has become yogurt cheese, combine it with remaining ingredients. Chill.

*1½ cups (approximately)*
*Calories per serving: 24 total; 0 fat; 0 sat-fat*

## FAUX GUACAMOLE

Your guests will never imagine that the dip they are eagerly devouring is made with asparagus. What a buy. A great-tasting treat at a cost of 0 fat calories.

2 tablespoons yogurt cheese*
1 pound asparagus
1 clove garlic, crushed
¼ teaspoon cayenne pepper
¼ teaspoon chili powder
1 tablespoon fresh lemon juice

2 ounces diced green chili
   peppers**
1 cup chopped tomatoes
1 tablespoon chopped onion
Whole-wheat pita bread

Prepare yogurt cheese a day in advance (see box).

Snap off bottom ends of asparagus and discard. Find a frying pan that will hold asparagus in one layer and fill it with an inch of water. Bring water to a boil and add asparagus. Cook until soft. Drain asparagus and purée with garlic in blender or food processor.

Mix in cayenne pepper, chili powder, lemon juice, yogurt cheese, chili peppers, tomatoes, and onion. Chill for several hours.

Serve with toasted whole-wheat pita pockets divided into quarters or Bagel Chips (recipe follows).

*1½ cups (approximately)*

| Calories | Total | Fat | Sat-fat |
|---|---|---|---|
| Per tablespoon | 7 | 0 | 0 |
| With pita bread quarter | 33 | 2 | 0 |

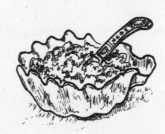

*See box on page 213.
**Available in small cans in most supermarkets

---

| **Yogurt Cheese** |
| :---: |

Yogurt cheese made with nonfat yogurt may be substituted for sour cream and cream cheese in some recipes, greatly reducing the sat-fat and total fat calories. It is easy to make. Place nonfat yogurt (without gelatin) in a coffee filter (or cheesecloth) in a coffeepot or in a strainer over a bowl. Cover and refrigerate overnight. As the yogurt drains, it condenses. Pour off whey and keep cheese in a covered container in the refrigerator. Add herbs, green onions, or Dijon mustard to make a flavored cheese.

*Calories per tablespoon: 7 total, 0 fat; 0 sat-fat*

---

# BAGEL CHIPS

A great crunchy snack — eat them alone or with dips.

Bagels (plain, onion, garlic, etc.)

### Flavor Options

1 clove garlic                    Cajun Seasoning Mix (page 51)
Chili powder                      Cinnamon and sugar

Preheat oven to 200°F.

Cut bagel into slices ¼–⅜ inch thick. They will look like very thin bagels. (Halve or quarter slices if you want smaller chips.) Place pieces on cookie sheet in one layer.

Either press garlic and spread over bagel slices, sprinkle chili powder or spice mix over them, leave them plain, or, for a sweet treat, sprinkle on a mix of cinnamon and sugar.

Bake for 1–2 hours.

*Calories per bagel chip: 38 total; 2 fat; 0 sat-fat*

# BABA GHANOUSH

| | |
|---|---|
| 1 medium eggplant | 1–2 cloves garlic |
| ¼ cup or more fresh lemon juice | ¼ cup chopped parsley |
| 3 tablespoons tahini (sesame seed paste)* | Salt to taste |

Peel eggplant, cut into bite-size pieces, and salt heavily. Set aside for 15 minutes. Rinse and squeeze eggplant and steam in vegetable steamer until soft.

Purée eggplant in food processor or blender.

Blend in lemon juice and tahini.

Just before serving, crush garlic into purée and mix in parsley and salt.

Taste. Add more lemon juice if you wish.

Serve with whole-wheat or plain pita bread cut into pieces.

*2 cups (approximately)*
*Calories per tablespoon: 12 total; 7 fat; 1 sat-fat*

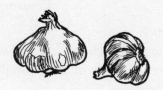

---

*Available at Mideastern food shops and many supermarkets.

## EGGPLANT APPETIZER

A tasty appetizer. Eat with quartered pita bread or crackers or heat and serve as a vegetable.

| | |
|---|---|
| 4 cups peeled, cubed eggplant | ½ cup Spanish olives |
| ½ cup chopped onion | ½ cup black olives |
| 4 cloves garlic, minced | 2 teaspoons capers |
| 2 stalks celery, sliced | 2 teaspoons brown sugar |
| 1 teaspoon olive oil | 2 tablespoons white vinegar |

Salt eggplant heavily and set aside for 15 minutes.

Rinse salt off eggplant under running water while squeezing out bitter juices.

Steam eggplant until tender.

Taste. If not bitter, set aside. If bitter, find a recipe without eggplant!

Sauté onion, garlic, and celery in olive oil until soft.

Mix in eggplant, olives, capers, brown sugar, and vinegar and heat until warm.

Eat hot, at room temperature, or chilled.

*10 servings*
*Calories per serving: 38 total; 24 fat; 5 sat-fat*

## SALSA

Salsa makes a lively addition to baked potatoes, Blackened Chicken (page 49), or Blackened Fish (page 108) and is a delicious dip.

| | |
|---|---|
| 2 pounds ripe tomatoes | 1 teaspoon cumin |
| ¼ cup chopped onion | 2 teaspoons chopped pickled |
| 2 cloves garlic, minced | jalapeño peppers |
| 2 tablespoons minced cilantro | 2 tablespoons fresh lime juice |

Roasting the tomatoes enhances their flavor. If you wish to roast them, cut them in half and place face down on a broiler pan close to the broiler coil. Broil for about 5 minutes or until they start to become charred and skin separates from tomato.

Cool slightly, remove skin, chop coarsely, drain, and place in medium bowl.

Mix in onion, garlic, cilantro, cumin, peppers, and lime juice.

Use warm or refrigerate.

*2 cups*
*Calories per tablespoon: 4 total; 0 fat; 0 sat-fat*

## CHICKPEA SANDWICH OR DIP

1 can (15 oz) chickpeas
2 cloves garlic
⅓ cup parsley
1 tablespoon tahini (sesame seed
   paste)*
Juice of 1 lemon (about ¼ cup)

4 six-inch whole-wheat pita
   bread pockets
Chopped tomatoes, green
   onions, and lettuce, for
   garnish

Drain chickpeas. Reserve liquid. In blender or food processor, chop garlic and parsley.

Add chickpeas, tahini, and lemon juice.

Blend until smooth, adding more chickpea liquid if spread is too stiff.

Make sandwiches by spooning chickpea spread into pita bread pockets.

Garnish with chopped tomatoes, green onions, and lettuce.

*4 sandwiches*

Use as a dip for vegetables, crackers, squares of pita, etc.

*1½ cups (approximately)*

| Calories | Total | Fat | Sat-fat |
|---|---|---|---|
| Per sandwich | 195 | 35 | 4 |
| Per tablespoon | 20 | 4 | 1 |

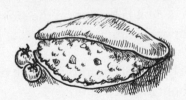

---

*Available at Mideastern food shops and many supermarkets.

## TED MUMMERY'S TURKEY BARBECUE

We discovered a most wonderful turkey barbecue while at a health conference in Steven's Point, Wisconsin. Ted Mummery, the owner of La Claire's Frozen Yogurt, Inc., has kindly allowed us to share his recipe with you. It's delicious in a whole-wheat pita pocket, on an onion bagel, or with any other bread.

| | |
|---|---|
| 5–6 pounds turkey breast | 1 heaping teaspoon garlic powder |
| 4 cans (14½ oz each) stewed tomatoes | 1½ heaping teaspoons onion powder |
| 2 large cans (12 oz each) tomato paste | 1 heaping teaspoon basil |
| 1 cup water | 1½ heaping teaspoons oregano |
| ½ cup brown sugar | 1 heaping teaspoon cayenne |
| ⅓ cup dark molasses | 1 teaspoon all-purpose seasoning |
| ½ cup apple cider vinegar | ½ teaspoon white pepper |
| 1 teaspoon hickory salt* (optional) or 1 teaspoon salt | |

Preheat oven to 350°F.

Remove skin and fat from turkey breast.

Bake turkey with breast down until fully cooked, about 1½–2½ hours. (You may do this the night before.) Refrigerate.

Mix tomatoes, tomato paste, and water in blender or food processor briefly. The tomatoes should be chopped, not puréed.

Place tomato mixture in 5-quart Crockpot or slow cooker. (You may also cook barbecue in a large pot on the stove.) Stir in remaining ingredients. Set Crockpot on automatic or cook at low heat for about 2 hours.

Pull turkey from bones and cut into bite-size pieces. Add turkey to sauce and cook for about another hour.

*30 half-cup servings*
*Calories per serving: 131 total; 5 fat; 1 sat-fat*

---

*Ted recommends 3 teaspoons of hickory salt. If you eat this barbecue often, I suggest eliminating the hickory salt, as it contains an unhealthy ingredient — smoke (charcoal).

## FROTHY FRUIT SHAKE

Use your imagination and the fruit you have in the house to create refreshing fruit shakes of different flavors. Here's one example:

1 cup strawberries
1 ripe banana, peeled and
    quartered
1 orange, peeled and halved

Dash of salt (optional)
½ cup crushed ice or 4–5 ice
    cubes

Place fruit and salt in a blender and purée.

Combine purée with ½ cup of finely crushed ice. You can make crushed ice by placing ice cubes in a plastic bag and smashing them with a meat-tenderizing mallet or hammer until crushed evenly. You can also crush ice in an electric ice-crusher. You may add ice cubes to the purée in the blender and blend until cubes are crushed.

*2 one-cup servings*
*Calories per serving: 105 total; 2 fat; 0 sat-fat*

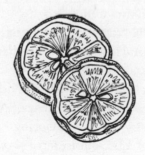

# ~10~
## Breads

STARCHES HAVE RECEIVED BAD PRESS over the years. Bread, rice, pasta, and potatoes have been associated with weight gain. Weight problems begin not with starch but with the fat that is put on the starch: bread slathered with margarine, potatoes stuffed with sour cream. An ounce of carbohydrate has less than *half* as many calories as an ounce of fat. An average piece of bread has 10 fat calories. Cover it with margarine and the fat calorie value goes up to 110.

You can cut down on fats by replacing fatty meats and high-fat dairy products with grains, potatoes, breads, and pasta. Many starchy foods (such as vegetables, whole grains, and potatoes with skin) provide fiber, bulk, vitamins, and minerals.

Many of the following recipes are for 1 loaf, so you can make them using your food processor. Double the ingredients for 2 loaves.

You can make any loaf into baguettes by following the recipe for French Bread, page 228, beginning with "Divide dough in half."

We have chosen to use olive oil in most of our breads because olive oil lowers LDL-cholesterol without lowering HDL-cholesterol. It also prevents the oxidation of LDL-cholesterol — the first step in the process of atherosclerosis. Choose a mild-tasting olive oil, and your taste buds won't notice the difference.

NOTE: The instruction "Let proof" means to wait for the yeast to ferment, swell, and get bubbly. This takes only a few minutes at most.

## ANADAMA BREAD

This version of the New England bread has whole-wheat flour added to make it healthier while retaining its wonderful taste and texture.

1 tablespoon active dry
   yeast
Pinch of sugar
¼ cup warm water
¾ cup cornmeal
1½ cups whole-wheat flour

1½ cups unbleached white flour
   (approximately)
1–1½ teaspoons salt
2 tablespoons olive oil
1 cup water
3 tablespoons molasses

Dissolve yeast with pinch of sugar in ¼ cup warm water in a large bowl or a food processor. Let proof.

Mix in cornmeal, whole-wheat flour, 1 cup of the white flour, and salt.

Stir in olive oil, 1 cup water, and molasses.

Knead dough for 10 minutes or process for 15 seconds or until dough is smooth and elastic, adding more white flour if necessary.

Place dough in a large oiled bowl, cover with a towel, and let rise in a warm place for 1 hour or until doubled in bulk.

From into a loaf and place in a loaf pan greased with margarine. Cover and let rise for 1 hour or until doubled in bulk.

Preheat oven to 400°F.

Bake loaf for 15 minutes.

Reduce heat to 350°F and bake about 30 minutes more or until loaf is golden brown and sounds hollow when tapped.

*1 loaf*

| Calories | Total | Fat | Sat-fat |
|---|---|---|---|
| Per ½-inch slice | 113 | 15 | 2 |
| Per loaf | 1919 | 257 | 42 |

# BUTTERMILK HERB BREAD

| | |
|---|---|
| 1 tablespoon active dry yeast | ¼ teaspoon oregano |
| 2 tablespoons sugar | ¼ teaspoon thyme |
| ¼ cup warm water | ½ cup nonfat buttermilk |
| 2–3 cups unbleached white flour | 2 tablespoons olive oil |
| 1 teaspoon salt | 1 egg |
| ¼ teaspoon marjoram | |

Place yeast, sugar, and water in a large bowl or in your food processor. Let proof.

Mix in 2 cups flour, salt, marjoram, oregano, and thyme.

Mix in buttermilk and olive oil. (If using a food processor, process at least 15 seconds.)

Mix in enough flour to make a stiff but soft dough.

Add egg. Knead dough for 10 minutes or process for 15 seconds or until dough is smooth and elastic.

Put dough in a large oiled bowl, cover with a towel, and let rise in a warm place for 1 hour or until doubled in bulk.

Form loaf and place in loaf pan greased with margarine. Cover and let rise 1 hour or until doubled in bulk.

Preheat oven to 375°F.

Bake loaf for about 35 minutes or until it is golden brown and sounds hollow when tapped.

*1 loaf*

| Calories | Total | Fat | Sat-fat |
|---|---|---|---|
| Per ½-inch slice | 108 | 18 | 3 |
| Per loaf | 1842 | 306 | 47 |

# CARDAMOM BREAD

| | |
|---|---|
| 1 tablespoon active dry yeast | 1 teaspoon salt |
| 2 tablespoons brown sugar | ¼–½ teaspoon cardamom* |
| ¼ cup warm water | 2 tablespoons olive oil |
| 2–4 cups unbleached white flour | 1 cup skim milk |

Combine yeast, brown sugar, and water in a large bowl or a food processor. Let proof.

Add 2 cups flour, salt, and cardamom and mix.

Mix in olive oil and skim milk. Add more flour until you produce a stiff dough.

Knead dough for 10 minutes or process for 15 seconds or until dough is smooth and elastic, adding more flour if necessary.

Place dough in a large oiled bowl, cover with a towel, and let rise in warm place for 1 hour or until doubled in bulk.

Roll into loaf and place in loaf pan greased with margarine.

Cover with a towel and let rise for 1 hour or until doubled in bulk.

Preheat oven to 425°F.

Bake loaf for 10 minutes.

Reduce heat to 350°F and bake for 30 minutes more or until loaf is golden brown and sounds hollow when tapped.

*1 loaf*
| Calories | Total | Fat | Sat-fat |
|---|---|---|---|
| Per ½-inch slice | 98 | 15 | 2 |
| Per loaf | 1663 | 255 | 41 |

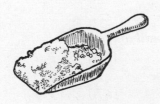

---

*For a totally different taste, substitute 1 teaspoon cinnamon.

# CHALLAH

A delicious bread for the Jewish Sabbath or just for enjoyable eating.

| | |
|---|---|
| 1 tablespoon active dry yeast | ½ teaspoon salt |
| 2 tablespoons sugar | 2 tablespoons olive oil |
| 1 cup warm water | 1 egg |
| 2–4 cups unbleached white flour | |

Place yeast, sugar, and ¼ cup warm water in a large bowl or a food processor. Let proof.

Mix in 2 cups flour and salt.

Add ¾ cup warm water, oil, and egg and mix or process for 15 seconds.

Knead dough for 10 minutes or process for 15 seconds or until dough is smooth and elastic, adding more flour if necessary.

Place dough in a large oiled bowl, cover with a towel, and let rise in warm place for 1 hour or until doubled in bulk.

Divide dough into two unequal portions, one-third and two-thirds.

Divide smaller portion of dough into three pieces. Roll each into a rope.

Divide larger portion into three pieces. Roll each into a rope.

Braid the three larger ropes and place on a greased cookie sheet.

Braid the three smaller ropes and place them on top of the larger braided pieces. Pinch the two braids together.

Cover with a towel and let rise for 1 hour or until doubled in bulk.

Preheat oven to 400°F.

Bake bread for 10 minutes.

Reduce heat to 375°F and bake for 30 minutes more or until golden brown.

*1 large loaf or 2 small loaves*

| Calories | Total | Fat | Sat-fat |
|---|---|---|---|
| Per ½-inch slice | 70 | 13 | 2 |
| Per loaf | 1670 | 317 | 47 |

# CINNAMON APPLESAUCE BREAD

| | |
|---|---|
| 1 tablespoon active dry yeast | 1 teaspoon cinnamon |
| 2 tablespoons brown sugar | ⅔ cup applesauce |
| 1 cup warm water | 1 tablespoon olive oil |
| 1½ cups whole-wheat flour | ½ apple, peeled, cored, and |
| 2 cups unbleached white flour | chopped (about ½ cup) |
| 1 teaspoon salt | ¼ cup raisins (optional) |

Combine yeast, sugar, and water in a large bowl or a food processor. Let proof.

Mix in whole-wheat flour, 1 cup of white flour, salt, and cinnamon.

Mix in applesauce and olive oil.

Add remaining cup of white flour and more of either or both flours until dough is fairly stiff. Knead dough for 10 minutes or process for 15 seconds or until dough is smooth and elastic, adding more flour if necessary.

Mix in apple and raisins.

Form dough into a ball. Place in an oiled bowl. Cover with towel and let rise for about 1 hour.

Roll dough into a loaf and place in loaf pan greased with margarine. Cover and let rise for an hour.

Preheat oven to 350°F. Bake for 50–60 minutes or until loaf sounds hollow when tapped.

*1 large loaf*

| Calories | Total | Fat | Sat-fat |
|---|---|---|---|
| Per ½-inch slice | 119 | 10 | 1 |
| Per loaf | 2025 | 177 | 24 |

# CRANBERRY BREAD

This tart but sweet loaf lies somewhere between bread and cake. To make sure you can bake it all year round, buy extra packages of cranberries at Thanksgiving and freeze them.

| | |
|---|---|
| 1½ cups cranberries | ¾ cup sugar |
| 2 cups unbleached white flour | ¾ cup orange juice |
| 1½ teaspoons baking powder | 1 tablespoon grated orange peel |
| ½ teaspoon baking soda | 2 tablespoons margarine |
| 1 teaspoon salt | 1 egg |

Preheat oven to 350°F and grease a loaf pan with margarine.

Chop cranberries in a food processor or hand chopper. Set aside.

In a large bowl, or the bowl of your electric mixer, combine flour, baking powder, baking soda, salt, and sugar.

Add orange juice, orange rind, margarine, and egg and mix until well blended.

Mix in cranberries.

Pour batter into loaf pan and bake for 45–55 minutes or until cake tester comes out clean.

*1 loaf*

| Calories | Total | Fat | Sat-fat |
|---|---|---|---|
| Per ½-inch slice | 112 | 15 | 3 |
| Per loaf | 1899 | 254 | 55 |

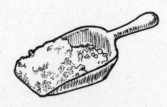

# CUMIN WHEAT BREAD

Although this is a totally whole-wheat bread, it is not the least bit heavy. It is a favorite with young children as well as adults.

| | |
|---|---|
| 1 tablespoon dry yeast | 1 teaspoon salt |
| ¼ cup warm water | ½ teaspoon whole cumin seeds |
| 2 tablespoons honey | 1½ tablespoons olive oil |
| 3½ cups whole-wheat flour | 1 cup skim milk |

In a large mixing bowl or the bowl of a food processor, combine yeast, water, and honey. Let proof.

Mix in 2 cups of the flour, salt, and cumin seeds.

Add oil and milk and mix or process well, adding more flour until dough is fairly stiff.

Knead dough 10 minutes or process for 15 seconds or until dough is smooth and elastic, adding more flour if necessary.

Form dough into a ball. Place in an oiled bowl. Cover and let rise for about 1 hour.

Roll dough into a loaf and place in loaf pan greased with margarine. Cover with towel and let rise for 1 hour.

Preheat oven to 375°F and bake for 50–60 minutes or until bread is golden and sounds hollow when tapped.

*1 loaf*

| Calories | Total | Fat | Sat-fat |
|---|---|---|---|
| Per ½-inch slice | 107 | 15 | 2 |
| Per loaf | 1814 | 252 | 35 |

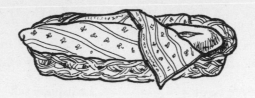

## FRENCH BREAD I

A French bread of peasant stock. Give yourself a treat and eat it warm, straight from the oven. It also freezes well. Make smaller loaves for submarine sandwiches. Any bread is an impressive gift to bring to friends. And this bread is so easy you'll be embarrassed to answer yes when asked if you made it yourself.

1½ tablespoons active dry yeast
½ teaspoon sugar
¼ cup warm water
2–3 cups unbleached white flour

1 teaspoon salt
2 tablespoons olive oil
1 cup water

Place yeast, sugar, and ¼ cup very warm, but *not hot,* water in a large bowl or a food processor. Let proof.

Mix in 2 cups flour and the salt.

Add olive oil and 1 cup water to flour and knead dough for 10 minutes or process for 15 seconds or until dough is smooth and elastic, adding more flour if necessary.

Place dough in large oiled bowl, cover with a towel, and let rise in a warm place for 1 hour or until doubled in bulk.

Divide dough in half.

Roll each half into a rectangle. Fold over in thirds like this:

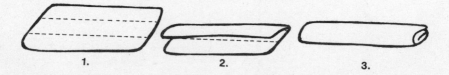

1.　　　　　2.　　　　　3.

Press the edge into dough after each fold.

Put into greased (with margarine) French bread pan that looks like this:

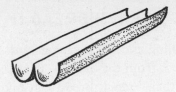

Cover and let rise for about 1 hour, or until doubled in bulk.
After 50 minutes, preheat oven to 450°F.
Uncover bread and slash with parallel or diagonal lines like this:

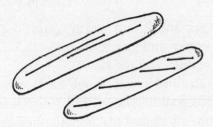

Place bread pan in oven on a diagonal to the right. For crustier loaves, put 4 ice cubes in bottom of oven to create steam.
In 5 minutes, add 4 more ice cubes.
In 10 minutes, shift pan so it is on a diagonal to the left, like this:

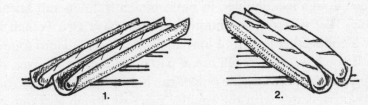

Reduce heat to 400°F and bake for 10 minutes more or until golden brown. Take loaves out of pan and cool or eat immediately.

Freezes nicely. If thawed, slice *before* reheating. Thawed French bread flakes like crazy when cut after reheating.

### 2 baguettes

| Calories | Total | Fat | Sat-fat |
|---|---|---|---|
| Per ½-inch slice | 87 | 13 | 2 |
| Per baguette | 874 | 133 | 19 |

# FRENCH BREAD II

There is almost nothing more satisfying and delicious than eating freshly baked bread hot from the oven — particularly French Bread II. This bread is lighter than French Bread I. It takes a long time to rise, but it's worth the wait.

1 tablespoon active dry yeast
1 tablespoon sugar
⅓ cup warm water

4+ cups unbleached white flour
1–1½ teaspoons salt
1¼ cups water

Place yeast, sugar, and ⅓ cup warm water in a large bowl or the bowl of a food processor and let proof.

Mix in 4 cups of flour and the salt.

Add 1¼ cups water and knead dough for 10 minutes or process for about 15 seconds. Keep adding flour until dough is smooth and elastic.

Make dough into a ball and place in an oiled bowl approximately twice the size of the dough so you'll be able to see when dough has doubled in size. Cover with a damp dish towel.

Place bowl in a warm place (on top of the refrigerator is often a nice, warm spot) and let rise until doubled in size. Dough will swell above edge of bowl. This will take at least 1½ hours.

When dough has doubled in bulk, punch it down and knead it a few times. Let it rest a few minutes. If you have two French bread pans, which together hold four loaves, divide the bread into four equal pieces. If you have one French bread pan that holds two loaves, divide the dough in half, then divide one of the halves in half again. You will make two baguettes with the smaller piece of dough and one round loaf with the larger piece.

For baguettes: Grease bread pan with margarine. Flatten dough into an oval. Squeeze dough into a long, thin rope with a diameter of about 1½ inches. Roll dough with the palms of both hands (to resemble the clay coils you made as a kid) to lengthen and smooth it. Place in bread pan.

For round bread: Grease bottom of an 8-inch cake pan with margarine. Form a ball by folding the edges of the dough under itself. Place in cake pan.

Cover bread with towel and let rise until baguette dough fills out pan.

When bread has completed its second rise (about 1½ hours), preheat oven to 450°F. Make 3 diagonal slashes in baguettes, about ⅛–⅜ inches deep. In round bread, make a 4-inch slash across center of the top. Make another slash through the center perpendicular to the first slash.

Place bread pans in oven. You will probably have to use two shelves or two ovens. Put 4 ice cubes on the oven floor to make the loaves crusty. Bake for 5 minutes. Add 4 more ice cubes. Bake for 5 more minutes. Shift direction of bread pans (see drawings on page 229) and bake for 10 more minutes or until golden brown.

### 4 baguettes, or 2 baguettes plus 1 round loaf

| Calories | Total | Fat | Sat-fat |
|---|---|---|---|
| Per baguette | 471 | 12 | 2 |
| Per 1½-inch slice | 52 | 1 | 0 |
| Per round loaf | 942 | 24 | 4 |
| Per ½-inch slice | 94 | 2 | 0 |

# FOCACCIA GENOVESE

| | |
|---|---|
| 1 package active dry yeast | 2¾ cups unbleached white flour |
| Pinch of sugar | 1 teaspoon olive oil |
| 1 cup warm water | 1 teaspoon or more garlic slivers |
| 2 teaspoons olive oil | 1 teaspoon rosemary |
| 1 teaspoon salt | ¼ teaspoon salt |

In a large bowl or food processor mix yeast, sugar, and water. Let proof.

Stir in 2 teaspoons olive oil, 1 teaspoon salt, and 2 cups flour. Process 15 seconds or mix until smooth, adding more flour until dough is smooth and firm. Place in bowl lightly oiled with olive oil and cover with towel for about 1 hour or until doubled in size.

Grease 12-inch-round pizza pan with olive oil. Punch down dough and spread evenly over pan. Cover with towel and let rise 30 minutes.

Preheat oven to 375°F.

Brush dough with 1 teaspoon olive oil. Distribute garlic slivers evenly over surface and push into dough. Sprinkle dough evenly with rosemary and ¼ teaspoon salt.

Bake dough 30 minutes or until golden.

*1 large flat loaf, 12 slices per loaf*

| Calories | Total | Fat | Sat-fat |
|---|---|---|---|
| Per slice | 116 | 13 | 2 |
| Per loaf | 1390 | 156 | 22 |

# GINGER-ORANGE BREAD

A very subtle taste of ginger pervades this whole-wheat bread.

1 tablespoon active dry yeast
2 tablespoons brown sugar
¼ cup warm water
1½ cups whole-wheat flour
1½ cups unbleached white flour
  (approximately)

1 teaspoon salt
2 teaspoons ground ginger
2 tablespoons olive oil
½ cup nonfat buttermilk
½ cup orange juice

Combine yeast, brown sugar, and warm water in a large bowl or a food processor. Let proof.

Mix in whole-wheat flour, white flour, salt, and ginger.

Add olive oil, buttermilk, and orange juice. Knead for 10 minutes or process for 15 seconds or until dough is smooth and elastic, adding more flour if necessary.

Place dough in a large oiled bowl, cover with a towel, and let rise in a warm place for 1 hour or until doubled in bulk.

Shape into a loaf and place in a loaf pan greased with margarine.

Cover with a towel and let rise in warm place for about 1 hour or until doubled in bulk.

Preheat oven to 400°F.

Bake loaf for 10 minutes.

Reduce heat to 350°F and bake for 30 minutes more or until golden brown.

*1 loaf*

| Calories | Total | Fat | Sat-fat |
|---|---|---|---|
| Per ½-inch slice | 99 | 16 | 3 |
| Per loaf | 1678 | 279 | 46 |

# HONEY WHOLE-WHEAT BREAD

Whole-grain breads are much more nutritious than breads made with white flour. In whole-grain flours, the entire kernel is ground, so vitamins, minerals, and fiber are not lost.

Honey Whole-Wheat Bread makes wonderful toast. Top it with bananas and cottage cheese and you have a filling, nutritious, and scrumptious breakfast. This bread freezes well.

This recipe makes four loaves of bread. Freeze the ones you are not using.

2 tablespoons active dry yeast

2 tablespoons salt

1 quart-size package nonfat dry milk

1 five-pound bag whole-wheat flour (about 16 cups)

6½ cups water

½ cup honey

½ cup olive oil

2 teaspoons cinnamon

½ teaspoon grated nutmeg

1½ cups rolled oats

½ cup raisins

In a mixing bowl, combine yeast, salt, nonfat dry milk, and 2 cups flour.

In a large saucepan, combine water, honey, and oil and heat until quite warm (about 115°F) but *not too hot* or you will kill the yeast.

Add liquid to dry ingredients in mixing bowl and beat for 4 minutes.

Mix in 4 cups flour.

Mix in cinnamon, nutmeg, oats, and raisins.

Keep adding flour until you produce a stiff dough. Your mixer probably will not be large enough to handle all the dough. When mixer reaches its limit, remove dough to a pastry board or counter and add flour until dough is stiff enough to knead.

Knead dough for 8–10 minutes or until smooth and elastic.

Place dough in large oiled bowl, cover with a towel, and let rise in warm place for about 1 hour or until doubled in bulk.

Form four loaves, place in loaf pans greased with margarine, cover with a towel, and let rise 1 hour or until doubled in bulk.

Preheat oven to 350°F.

Bake loaves for 45 minutes to 1 hour or until they are golden brown and sound hollow when tapped.

*4 loaves*

| Calories | Total | Fat | Sat-fat |
|---|---|---|---|
| Per ½-inch slice | 130 | 17 | 2 |
| Per loaf | 2222 | 342 | 39 |

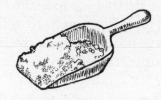

# MULTI-GRAIN BREAD

This bread has a wonderful, nutty taste, smells delicious while it is baking, and is healthy. What more could you ask?

½ cup rolled oats
1 tablespoon dry yeast
¼ cup warm water
2 tablespoons honey
6+ cups whole-wheat flour
½ cup unbleached white flour
¼ cup wheat germ

1 teaspoon salt
1 tablespoon olive oil
2 cups skim milk
1 cup water
½ teaspoon olive oil to grease
  bowl

Spread rolled oats on the tray of a toaster oven or on a cookie sheet and bake at 350°F until toasted, about 5–10 minutes. Set aside.

Meanwhile, in a large mixing bowl or the bowl of a food processor, combine yeast, ¼ cup water, and honey. Let proof (yeast becomes bubbly).

Add 2 cups of whole-wheat flour, the white flour, wheat germ, salt, and oats and mix.

Add olive oil, milk, and water and mix. Add more flour until dough is fairly stiff.

Knead dough for 10 minutes or process for 15 seconds or until dough is smooth and elastic, adding more flour as necessary.

Form dough into a ball and place in oiled bowl. Cover with a towel and let rise for 1 hour.

Grease a loaf pan with margarine or cooking spray.

Roll dough into a loaf and place in loaf pan. Cover with a towel and let rise for 1 hour.

Preheat oven to 350°F and bake bread for 60–75 minutes or until it is golden and sounds hollow when tapped.

*1 loaf, 20 slices*

| | Calories Total | Fat | Sat-fat |
|---|---|---|---|
| Per slice | 159 | 9 | 0 |
| Per loaf | 3178 | 188 | 5 |

## OATMEAL BREAD

| | |
|---|---|
| 1 cup water | 1 tablespoon active dry yeast |
| 1 cup rolled oats | Pinch of sugar |
| 2 tablespoons honey | ⅓ cup warm water |
| 1 tablespoon olive oil | 2½ cups unbleached white flour |
| 1 teaspoon salt | (approximately) |

In a small saucepan, boil 1 cup water and add oats, honey, oil, and salt. Let cool.

Combine yeast, sugar, and ⅓ cup warm water in a large bowl or a food processor. Let proof.

Add 2 cups flour to the yeast mixture.

When oat mixture is warm, but *not hot,* add it to the flour mixture and knead dough 10 minutes or process 15 seconds or until dough is smooth and elastic, adding more flour if necessary.

Place dough in a large oiled bowl, cover with a towel, and let rise in a warm place for 1 hour or until doubled in bulk.

Form dough into a loaf and place in a loaf pan greased with margarine. Cover and let rise about 1 hour or until doubled in bulk.

Preheat oven to 350°F.

Bake for 45 minutes or until golden brown.

*1 loaf*

| Calories | Total | Fat | Sat-fat |
|---|---|---|---|
| Per ½-inch slice | 96 | 11 | 2 |
| Per loaf | 1630 | 196 | 31 |

# ONION FLAT BREAD

Easy and a great treat!

| | |
|---|---|
| 1 tablespoon active dry yeast | 1 teaspoon + a few shakes salt |
| 1 pinch sugar | 1 teaspoon olive oil |
| 1 cup warm water | 1 cup chopped onion |
| 2½–3 cups unbleached white flour* | 1 teaspoon paprika |

Place yeast, sugar, and water in large bowl or a food processor. Let proof.

Mix in 2 cups flour and salt. Knead for 10 minutes or process for 15 seconds or until smooth and elastic, adding flour if necessary.

Place dough in an oiled bowl, cover with a towel, and let rise in a warm place for an hour or until doubled in bulk.

Punch dough down and split in half. Let rest for 5 minutes.

Meanwhile, grease two 9-inch cake pans with margarine.

Press dough into cake pans.

Spread olive oil over tops and press onions into surface.

Let rise about 45 minutes or until doubled in bulk.

Preheat oven to 450°F.

Sprinkle tops with paprika and a few shakes of salt.

Bake 20–25 minutes, until lightly browned.

*2 loaves, 8 slices per loaf*

| Calories | Total | Fat | Sat-fat |
|---|---|---|---|
| Per slice | 83 | 4 | 0 |
| Per loaf | 667 | 32 | 3 |

---

*For a slightly different taste, use 1 cup of whole-wheat flour along with 1½–2 cups unbleached white flour.

# PUMPERNICKEL BREAD

1 tablespoon yeast

¼ cup warm water

Pinch of sugar

1 cup rye flour

2 cups whole-wheat flour
  (approximately)

2 cups unbleached white flour

1 teaspoon salt

2 tablespoons olive oil

2 tablespoons molasses

1¼ cups warm water

1 tablespoon caraway seeds

Corn flour

Place yeast in a large bowl or a food processor. Add ¼ cup warm water and sugar. Let proof.

Mix in rye flour, whole-wheat flour, 1½ cups white flour, and salt.

Add olive oil, molasses, and 1¼ cups warm water. Knead for 10 minutes or process for 15 seconds or until dough is smooth and elastic, adding more white flour if necessary.

Knead in caraway seeds.

Place dough in a large oiled bowl, cover with a towel, and let rise in a warm place for 1 hour or until doubled in bulk.

Sprinkle corn flour on a baking sheet.

Form dough into a round or loaf, place on baking sheet, cover, and let rise 1 hour or until doubled in bulk.

Preheat oven to 450°F.

Bake loaf for 10 minutes.

Reduce heat to 350°F and bake for 35 minutes more or until loaf sounds hollow when tapped.

*1 large loaf*

| Calories | Total | Fat | Sat-fat |
|---|---|---|---|
| Per ½-inch slice | 92 | 12 | 2 |
| Per loaf | 2273 | 301 | 39 |

## SHAKER DAILY LOAF

1 tablespoon active dry yeast
Pinch of sugar
¼ cup warm water
6 cups unbleached white flour
    (approximately)

2¼ cups skim milk
2 tablespoons margarine
2 tablespoons maple syrup or
    honey
2 teaspoons salt

Dissolve yeast and sugar in warm water in a large bowl or a food processor. Let proof (become bubbly).

Mix in 3 cups of the flour.

In a small saucepan, scald skim milk. Remove from heat.

Add margarine, maple syrup, and salt to milk and mix until margarine melts.

When liquid has cooled to lukewarm, add to flour in bowl.

Stir in more flour, ½ cup at a time, until dough is fairly stiff.

Knead dough for 10 minutes or process for 15 seconds or until dough is smooth and elastic.

Place dough in a large oiled bowl, cover with a towel, and let rise in a warm place for 1 hour or until doubled in bulk.

Remove dough from bowl and divide it in half.

Let dough rest, covered, for 10 minutes.

Roll into two loaves and place in loaf pans greased with margarine.

Cover and let rise until doubled (1–2 hours).

Preheat oven to 350°F.

Bake loaves for 35–40 minutes or until they are golden brown and sound hollow when tapped.

*2 loaves*

| Calories | Total | Fat | Sat-fat |
|---|---|---|---|
| Per ½-inch slice | 90 | 7 | 2 |
| Per loaf | 1512 | 117 | 28 |

# WHOLE-WHEAT BANANA RAISIN BREAD

This is a banana bread, not a banana cake. It is dense and delicious.

1 tablespoon yeast
Pinch of sugar
¼ cup warm water
1 cup unbleached white flour
2½ cups whole-wheat flour
1 teaspoon salt

2 ripe bananas, mashed
2 tablespoons molasses
1 tablespoon olive oil
1 cup nonfat buttermilk
¼ cup raisins (optional)

Combine yeast, sugar, and water in a large bowl or the bowl of a food processor. Let proof.

Mix in white flour, 2 cups of whole-wheat flour, and salt.

Mix bananas, molasses, oil, and buttermilk together and add to the flours. Add more whole-wheat flour to make a dough you can knead.

Knead for 10 minutes or process for 15 seconds or until dough is smooth and elastic, adding more whole-wheat flour if necessary.

Add raisins.

Place dough in a large oiled bowl. Rotate dough to cover surface with a film of olive oil. Cover bowl with a towel and let rise in a warm place for about 1 hour or until doubled in bulk.

Form loaf and place in a loaf pan greased with margarine. Cover with a towel and let rise in a warm place for about 1 hour or until doubled in bulk.

Preheat oven to 350°F.

Bake for 45–55 minutes or until golden brown and hollow when tapped.

*1 large loaf*

| Calories | Total | Fat | Sat-fat |
|---|---|---|---|
| Per ½-inch slice | 123 | 11 | 2 |
| Per loaf | 2099 | 195 | 30 |

## WHOLE-WHEAT BAGELS

1 tablespoon active dry yeast     1½ cups unbleached white flour
3 tablespoons sugar                1 teaspoon salt
1 cup warm water                   2 tablespoons olive oil
1½ cups whole-wheat flour

Mix yeast, sugar, and warm water in a large bowl or a food processor. Let proof.

Mix in whole-wheat flour, white flour, and salt.

Knead for 8–10 minutes or process for 15 seconds or until dough is smooth and elastic, adding more flour if necessary.

Place dough in a large oiled bowl, cover with a towel, and let rise in a warm place for 40 minutes. Punch down.

Divide dough into 12 pieces. Roll each piece into tube about 5 inches long and ¾ inch wide. Pinch into a circle to make a bagel.

Preheat oven to 350°F and grease cookie sheet with oil.

Fill a medium saucepan with water. Add olive oil and bring to a boil.

Drop a bagel into the boiling water.

When it rises to the top, remove it with a slotted spoon or spatula so excess water can drip off.

Repeat this process with the rest of the bagels.

Place bagels on cookie sheet and bake for 10 minutes.

Raise heat to 400°F and bake for 10 minutes more.

*12 bagels*
*Calories per bagel: 115 total; 23 fat; 1 sat-fat*

# SESAME BREADSTICKS

Beware! These breadsticks are habit-forming.

1 teaspoon active dry yeast
¼ cup warm water
⅔ cup whole-wheat flour
2 or more cups unbleached
   white flour
1 teaspoon salt, optional

⅔ cup nonfat skim milk
1 tablespoon olive oil
1 egg white
2 teaspoons water
1 tablespoon sesame seeds

Place yeast and warm water in large bowl or a food processor. Let proof.

Mix in flours and salt.

Add milk and olive oil and knead for 10 minutes or process for 15 seconds or until dough is smooth and elastic, adding more flour if necessary.

Place dough in ungreased bowl, cover with a towel, and let rise 1 hour.

Preheat oven to 400°F.

On a lightly floured surface, roll dough into a ¼-inch-thick rectangle. One dimension of the rectangle should be the length of your breadsticks.

Cut the dough into ½-inch strips. (If you prefer thicker breadsticks, cut the dough into 1-inch strips.)

Roll each strip in your palms to make a breadstick and lay it on an ungreased baking sheet. Place sticks in a row about ½ inch apart.

Beat egg white and water together and brush onto breadsticks.

Sprinkle sesame seeds evenly over breadsticks.

Count breadsticks so you can calculate their sat-fat calories.

Bake for 20–30 minutes or until golden brown. Cool on a rack.

*35 six-inch sticks (approximately)*
*Calories for entire recipe: 1423 total; 196 fat; 30 sat-fat*
*Calories per breadstick: 41 total; 6 fat; 1 sat-fat*

## BRAN MUFFINS

Wheat bran, made from the outer coverings of wheat kernels, is rich in vitamins, minerals, and insoluble dietary fiber. Insoluble dietary fiber promotes regularity and is believed to protect against colon cancer.

| | |
|---|---|
| 1 cup whole-wheat flour | 1 cup nonfat buttermilk |
| 1 cup wheat bran | 1 egg, beaten |
| 3 tablespoons brown sugar | 3 tablespoons molasses |
| ¼ teaspoon salt | 2 tablespoons olive oil |
| 1 teaspoon baking soda | ⅓ cup raisins |
| ½ teaspoon baking powder | |

Preheat oven to 400°F. Grease a 12-cup muffin tin with margarine.

Combine whole-wheat flour, wheat bran, brown sugar, salt, baking soda, and baking powder. Set aside.

In a mixing bowl, mix buttermilk, egg, molasses, and oil.

Add dry ingredients and mix until just moistened.

Fold in raisins.

Fill cups of muffin tin and bake for about 15 minutes or until muffins are golden brown and a cake tester comes out clean.

*12 muffins*
*Calories per muffin: 116 total; 23 fat; 4 sat-fat*

# GINGERBREAD MUFFINS

These muffins taste like cake.

| | |
|---|---|
| 1 cup unbleached white flour | ¼ teaspoon allspice |
| ¾ cup whole-wheat flour | ¼ teaspoon grated nutmeg |
| ¼ cup sugar | ¾ cup nonfat buttermilk |
| ¼ cup brown sugar | ⅓ cup applesauce |
| 1 teaspoon baking soda | 1 egg |
| ¼ teaspoon salt | 1 egg white |
| 1 teaspoon ginger | ¼ cup light unsulphured |
| 1 teaspoon cinnamon |    molasses |
| ¼ teaspoon cloves | |

Preheat oven to 400°F and grease a 12-cup muffin tin with margarine.

Combine flours, sugars, baking soda, salt, and spices in a large bowl. Set aside.

In a large mixing bowl, combine buttermilk, applesauce, egg, egg white, and molasses.

Add flour mixture to buttermilk mixture. Do not overmix.

Pour into cups of muffin tin and bake for 15 minutes, or until cake tester comes out clean.

*12 muffins*
*Calories per muffin: 124 total; 6 fat; 1 sat-fat*

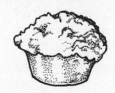

### Oat Bran

Oat bran, a food rich in soluble fiber, has a modest effect on lowering blood cholesterol levels.

## MOTHER'S OAT BRAN MUFFINS

2¼ cups oat bran
¼ cup brown sugar
¼ cup chopped walnuts
¼ cup raisins
1 tablespoon baking powder

½ teaspoon salt
¾ cup skim milk
1 egg + 1 egg white, beaten
¼ cup honey
¼ cup applesauce

Preheat oven to 425°F. Grease a 12-cup muffin tin with margarine.

Combine oat bran, brown sugar, walnuts, raisins, baking powder, and salt.

Add skim milk, eggs, honey, and applesauce. Mix until ingredients are just moistened.

Fill cups of muffin tin and bake for 15 minutes or until muffins are golden brown and a cake tester comes out clean.

Cool in muffin tin before removing.

*12 muffins*

| Calories per muffin | Total | Fat | Sat-fat |
|---|---|---|---|
| | 140 | 30 | 3 |
| Without walnuts | 126 | 15 | 1 |

# APRICOT OAT BRAN MUFFINS

Healthy and delicious — a good snack or breakfast on the run.

½ cup orange juice
1 cup dried apricots, chopped
  (easily done in food
  processor)
¼ cup brown sugar
1 cup oat bran
¼ cup wheat germ

¾ cup whole-wheat flour
1 teaspoon baking powder
1 teaspoon baking soda
2 tablespoons applesauce
½ cup skim milk
1 egg

Preheat oven to 400°F. Grease a 12-cup muffin tin with margarine.

In a small saucepan, heat orange juice until boiling. Mix in apricots and brown sugar.

Remove saucepan from heat and cool apricot mixture slightly.

In a medium bowl, combine oat bran, wheat germ, whole-wheat flour, and baking powder. Set aside.

In a mixing bowl, beat together applesauce, skim milk, and egg.

Add dry ingredients and apricot–orange juice mixture to milk mixture and mix until just moistened.

Fill cups of muffin tin and bake for 15 minutes or until muffins are golden brown and a cake tester comes out clean.

*12 muffins*
*Calories per muffin: 114 total; 10 fat; 1 sat-fat*

## BUTTERMILK PANCAKES

Breakfast need not be a problem for those watching their fat intake. In addition to the preceding bread and muffin recipes, try these pancakes and waffles.

Instead of using sour cream (493 fat calories per cup) or whole milk (75 fat calories per cup), make your pancakes with nonfat buttermilk (0 fat calories per cup). Buttermilk enhances the taste of waffles and pancakes. These delicious pancakes will hardly make a dent in your Fat Budget.

Use maple syrup or powdered sugar to sweeten pancakes and waffles. Butter adds only unneeded fat.

HINT: Use a cast-iron griddle, and you will need little or no margarine to keep your pancakes from sticking to the surface.

½ cup unbleached white flour
¼ cup whole-wheat flour
½ teaspoon baking powder
½ teaspoon baking soda
½ cup nonfat buttermilk*

¼–½ cup skim milk*
1 egg white, lightly beaten
2 teaspoons olive oil (optional)
Margarine to grease grill

In a large bowl, combine the flours, baking powder, and baking soda.

Mix in buttermilk and skim milk, egg white, and oil. Do not overmix.

*Lightly* grease a hot griddle or skillet with margarine, making sure you keep track of the amount you use.

For each pancake, spread a tablespoon of batter on griddle. When pancake solidifies and edges come away from griddle, turn the pancake. The bottom should be golden brown. Cook until other side is also golden.

*16 pancakes (approximately)*

---

*For equally delicious pancakes, substitute ½ cup nonfat yogurt for the ½ cup nonfat buttermilk.

| Calories | Total | Fat | Sat-fat |
|---|---|---|---|
| Total batter | 495 | 90 | 13 |
| Per pancake | 31 | 13 | 1 |
| With no added oil | | | |
| Total batter | 415 | 10 | 1 |
| Per pancake | 26 | 1 | 0 |

If you used more than 1 teaspoon of margarine to grease your griddle, for each pancake add 6 total calories, 6 fat calories, and 1 sat-fat calorie for each additional teaspoon.

# BUTTERMILK WAFFLES

| | |
|---|---|
| 1 egg white at room temperature | ½ teaspoon salt |
| 1 cup whole-wheat flour | 1 cup buttermilk |
| 1 cup unbleached white flour | 1 cup skim milk |
| 2 teaspoons baking powder | 2 teaspoons olive oil |

Spray waffle iron with cooking spray and preheat.

In a medium bowl, combine whole-wheat flour, white flour, baking powder, and salt.

Add buttermilk and skim milk. *Do not overmix.*

Fold in egg white and oil.

Place batter on waffle iron in amounts specified by your waffle-iron instructions. Cook accordingly.

*5 waffles*

| Calories | Total | Fat | Sat-fat |
|---|---|---|---|
| Total batter | 1102 | 107 | 16 |
| Per square* | 220 | 21 | 3 |

---

*Because waffle irons come in many sizes, this recipe may make more or less than 5 waffle squares. Divide 1102 by the number of waffle squares you make to figure out the total calories per square (for example, 1102 ÷ 5 = 220). Divide 107 by the number of waffle squares to figure out the fat calories per square (for example, 107 ÷ 5 = 21). Divide 16 by the number of waffle squares to figure out the sat-fat calories per square (for example, 16 ÷ 5 = 3).

# CINNAMON FRENCH TOAST

2 egg whites
3 tablespoons skim milk
½ teaspoon vanilla
½ teaspoon ground cinnamon
Pinch of grated nutmeg

3 slices whole-wheat bread or
   French bread
2 teaspoons margarine
   (optional)

In a shallow dish, mix egg whites, skim milk, vanilla, cinnamon, and nutmeg.

Soak both sides of bread in mixture.

Heat a large frying pan or cast-iron griddle.* Spread margarine over it if necessary.

Add bread. Reduce heat to medium.

Turn bread after 2 minutes. Cook until golden brown and crispy.

*3 servings*

| Calories | Total | Fat | Sat-fat |
|---|---|---|---|
| Without margarine | 75 | 6 | 0 |
| With margarine | 95 | 26 | 4 |

---

*Use a cast-iron griddle, which requires little or no margarine to keep the French toast from sticking, to reduce the sat-fat and total fat even more.

# ~11~
# Desserts

**YOU MIGHT THINK DESSERT** would be the most difficult part of the meal to make low in fat. This is not true. There are many desserts that not only are scrumptious and beautiful but fit perfectly into a low-fat diet.

The trick to keeping desserts low in fat is to substitute nonfat yogurt, nonfat buttermilk, or skim milk for sour cream, sweet cream, or whole milk, and try substituting applesauce for butter, margarine, or oil. Reduce eggs to no more than one, and substitute egg whites for additional eggs.

You may be surprised that we use olive oil in making some of these desserts. Olive oil is the oil of choice because it lowers LDL-cholesterol without lowering HDL-cholesterol. Try using a mild-tasting olive oil in your baked goods. Only your arteries will be able to detect a difference.

But, whether high in fat, low in fat, or even nonfat, desserts are full of empty sugar calories and should be saved for splurges.

NOTE: You will notice that we recommend grated nutmeg in many recipes. Buy whole nutmegs at your grocery store and simply grate one when you need nutmeg in a recipe. The advantage is that each time you grate one it is fresh and thus has the taste it is supposed to have.

We recommend unbleached white flour because when a flour is bleached, it loses many of its important nutritional qualities.

If your cookie sheet has a raised rim, turn it over and use the bottom. The flat surface will make it easier to remove cookies, meringues, etc.

# APPLE CAKE

A moist, hearty cake that is easy to make.

¾ cup brown sugar
½ cup applesauce
1 teaspoon vanilla
1 egg
1 egg white
¾ cup unbleached white flour
1 cup whole-wheat flour

½ teaspoon salt
1 teaspoon baking soda
1½ teaspoons cinnamon
¼ teaspoon grated nutmeg
4 cups Delicious apples, peeled
    and cut into chunks

Preheat oven to 350°F. Grease an 8-inch springform pan with margarine and dust with flour.

In an electric mixer, beat together brown sugar and applesauce.

Add vanilla, egg, and egg white and beat until smooth.

Add flours, salt, baking soda, cinnamon, and nutmeg and beat until smooth.

With a large (wooden) spoon or rubber spatula, mix in apples. The batter will be *very* sticky and stiff.

Spoon batter into pan and bake for 40–60 minutes or until a cake tester comes out clean.

*10 slices*
*Calories per slice: 189 total; 6 fat; 2 sat-fat*

# TANTE NANCY'S APPLE CRUMB CAKE

Apple Crumb Cake is luscious. The crust is thick, crunchy, and sweet. The slightly tart apples melt in your mouth. This cake also tastes divine with peaches or blueberries or a combination of the two.

2–2½ pounds tart apples (about 6–7 large), peeled, cored, and sliced

⅓ cup water

¼ cup sugar

2 cups unbleached white flour

¾ cup sugar

1½ teaspoons baking powder

½ cup margarine

1 egg yolk

Preheat oven to 350°F. Grease an 8-inch springform pan with margarine.

In a large pot, cook apple slices with water and ¼ cup sugar until apples are tender but not mushy. Drain and reserve.

In a small bowl, mix flour, ¾ cup sugar, and baking powder.

With a pastry blender, cut in margarine.

Cut in egg yolk.

Reserve 1 cup of flour mixture for topping. Press remainder into bottom and sides of pan.

Spoon drained apples into pan.

Cover with reserved topping.

Bake for about 1 hour or until crust is golden brown.

*12 slices*
*Calories per slice: 220 total; 60 fat; 14 sat-fat*

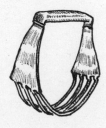

# BANANA CAKE

This Banana Cake is out of the ordinary. Rich and full-bodied.

1 cup whole-wheat flour
½ cup unbleached white flour
¼ cup wheat germ
1 teaspoon cinnamon
½ teaspoon grated nutmeg
2 teaspoons baking powder
¼ teaspoon baking soda

¼ teaspoon salt
½ cup applesauce
½ cup brown sugar
¾ teaspoon vanilla
1 egg
3 ripe bananas, mashed
5 prunes, chopped

Preheat oven to 350°F. Grease a loaf pan with margarine.

Mix flours, wheat germ, cinnamon, nutmeg, baking powder, baking soda, and salt and set aside.

In an electric mixer, mix applesauce and brown sugar. Add vanilla and egg and mix well.

Add bananas and blend until smooth. Mix in flour mixture.

Fold in prunes.

Pour batter into loaf pan and bake for 40–60 minutes or until a cake tester comes out clean.

*10 slices*
*Calories per slice: 166 total; 6 fat; 2 sat-fat*

# THE YORK BLUEBERRY CAKE

½ cup brown sugar
1 teaspoon cinnamon
2 cups unbleached white flour
1 teaspoon baking soda
½ teaspoon salt
2 cups blueberries

½ cup applesauce
¾ cup sugar
1 egg
2 egg whites
1 cup nonfat yogurt
1 teaspoon vanilla

Preheat oven to 350°F and grease a 13×9-inch baking pan with margarine.

Combine brown sugar and cinnamon and set aside.

In a large bowl, combine flour, baking soda, and salt.

Mix ¼ cup of flour mixture with blueberries and set aside.

In a large mixing bowl, mix applesauce and sugar.

Beat in eggs and egg whites.

Stir in yogurt and vanilla.

Add remaining flour to batter and beat until smooth.

Stir in floured blueberries.

Spread half of batter into baking pan and sprinkle half of brown sugar mixture over it.

Cover with remaining batter (it will barely cover the entire surface) and top with remaining brown sugar mixture.

Bake for 30–45 minutes or until cake tester comes out clean.

*20 squares*
*Calories per square: 113 total; 3 fat; 1 sat-fat*

# DIVINE BUTTERMILK POUND CAKE

You will not believe how light and fine-grained this cake is.

| | |
|---|---|
| 1¾ cups cake flour | ¾ cup sugar |
| ½ teaspoon baking soda | 1 egg + 2 egg whites |
| 1 teaspoon baking powder | ½ teaspoon vanilla |
| ¼ teaspoon salt | ¼ teaspoon almond extract |
| ½ cup margarine | ¾ cup nonfat buttermilk |

Preheat oven to 375°F and grease an 8-inch springform pan with margarine.

Combine flour, baking soda, baking powder, and salt and set aside.

In an electric mixer, cream margarine and sugar.

Add egg and egg whites, vanilla, and almond extract and mix until smooth.

Add flour mixture and buttermilk and mix until smooth.

Pour into springform pan and bake for 30–40 minutes or until cake tester comes out clean.

When cool, frost it with our number-one favorite choice, Don Mauer's Fantastic Fudge Frosting (page 262).

*12 slices*

| *Calories per slice:* | *Total* | *Fat* | *Sat-fat* |
|---|---|---|---|
| | 180 | 64 | 13 |
| With Don Mauer's Frosting | 245 | 68 | 13 |

# CARROT CAKE WITH CREAM CHEESE ICING

2⅔ cups grated carrots (not
  packed down)
⅔ cup crushed pineapple
⅓ cup apple butter
¾ cup sugar
3 egg whites

1½ teaspoons vanilla
1⅓ cups flour
1¾ teaspoons baking soda
1¾ teaspoons cinnamon
½ teaspoon salt
½ cup raisins

### Cream Cheese Icing

4 oz fat-free cream cheese
3 tablespoons powdered sugar

½ teaspoon vanilla

### The Cake

Preheat oven to 375°F. Grease an 8×8-inch baking pan with margarine or a cooking spray.

In a large bowl, combine carrots, pineapple, apple butter, sugar, egg whites, and vanilla. Stir until well blended.

Add flour, baking soda, cinnamon, and salt. Blend well.

Stir in raisins.

Spread batter in pan. Bake for 35 minutes or until cake tester comes out clean.

Cool. Make icing.

### The Icing

In a food processor or mixer, process or beat cream cheese, sugar, and vanilla until very smooth. Scrape sides and bottom and process again. There should not be any lumps.

Spread icing over top of cake.

*16 squares*
*Calories per square: 111 total; 0 fat; 0 sat-fat*
*Calories per iced square: 122 total; 0 fat; 0 sat-fat*

# CHEESECAKE!

I never believed you could make a cheesecake low in fat. With this recipe I have become a believer. While not *exactly* the same as real cheesecake, this low-fat version is delicious.

NOTE: Start this cake more than a day in advance because it takes 24 hours to make the yogurt cheese, and the cake must chill for a few hours after you bake it.

Yogurt Cheese (page 213), made from two 32-ounce containers vanilla nonfat yogurt

Graham Cracker Crust* (page 280), made with 1 tablespoon or no margarine

### Filling

Yogurt Cheese
½ cup sugar

2 tablespoons cornstarch
5 egg whites

The day before you plan to serve the cheesecake, prepare the yogurt cheese. But drain the yogurt for a full 24 hours to create a cheesecake consistency.

When yogurt cheese is ready, prepare Graham Cracker Crust in a 9-inch pie plate.

Preheat oven to 325°F.

Place yogurt cheese in a large bowl.

In a small bowl, mix sugar and cornstarch together, then add to yogurt cheese. Blend.

Mix in egg whites. Blend well, but do not beat air into batter.

Pour batter into crust and bake for about 60–70 minutes or until center is set. Cool slightly, then refrigerate until chilled. You may top with fruit topping.

### 12 slices

| Calories per slice: | Total | Fat | Sat-fat |
|---|---|---|---|
| With crust made with 1 tablespoon margarine | 120 | 16 | 4 |
| With crust made with no fat | 112 | 8 | 3 |

---

*If you use a commercial crust, divide total, fat, and sat-fat calories of crust by 12 and add to filling (70 total calories/slice and no fat) to determine amounts per slice.

# LEMON CHEESECAKE

Cheesecake doesn't have to be packed with fat to be good. This delectable light cake is simple to make, low-low-low in fat, and delicious.

Zest* of 1 lemon, chopped
3 egg whites
⅔ cup sugar
¼ cup cornstarch
¼ teaspoon vanilla

2⅔ cup low-fat (1%) cottage cheese
8 low-fat 2-inch×2-inch graham crackers** to make ⅔ cup graham cracker crumbs

Preheat oven to 325°F and grease an 8-inch springform pan with margarine. You will also need an ovenproof pan large enough to hold the springform pan.

Fill a pot or teakettle with water and start heating it to a boil.

Place lemon zest, egg whites, sugar, cornstarch, vanilla, and cottage cheese in a blender and blend until very, very smooth (no lumps). Pour into springform pan.

Place springform pan in the middle of the larger pan.

*Carefully* pour boiling water into large pan so it reaches about halfway up the sides of the springform pan.

Bake for 60 minutes or until cheesecake is set and cake tester comes out clean.

Remove pan from water and refrigerate cake in pan for at least 4 hours or overnight. It should be really cold.

In a food processor, turn graham crackers into ⅔ cup fine crumbs. After cheesecake has been refrigerated for 4 or more hours, spread crumbs evenly over cake surface and gently pat them down. You may do this just before serving. Before serving, carefully run knife around edge of springform pan and remove sides.

*8 slices*
*Calories per slice: 160 total; 10 fat; 3 sat-fat*

---

*The yellow part of the lemon peel is called the zest. You can use a zester to remove the zest, then chop it in a mini-chopper or food processor or by hand. You can also grate the lemon with a hand grater.
**Use commercial low-fat graham crackers or make Honey Graham Crackers (page 292).

## DON MAUER'S DELECTABLE
## CHOCOLATE CAKE

Don Mauer, a Choose to Lose success story, lost 103 pounds and went on to create his own recipes and become a cookbook author. He has given us permission to print this scrumptious low-fat chocolate cake recipe from *Lean and Lovin' It*.

### Cake

2 teaspoons Dutch-process
  unsweetened cocoa powder
1 cup unbleached white flour
⅓ cup + 1 tablespoon Dutch-
  process unsweetened cocoa
  powder
1 teaspoon baking powder

1 teaspoon baking soda
6 large egg whites, at room
  temperature
1⅓ cups firmly packed dark
  brown sugar
1 cup nonfat yogurt
1 teaspoon vanilla

### Topping

1 tablespoon Dutch-process
  unsweetened cocoa powder

1 tablespoon powdered sugar

Set oven rack in middle of oven and preheat to 350°F. Lightly spray bottom and sides of an 8-inch high-sided springform pan with olive or canola oil. Dust bottom and sides of pan with 2 teaspoons cocoa powder; tap out excess. Set aside.

In a medium mixing bowl, whisk or stir flour, cocoa, baking powder, and baking soda together, about 30 seconds. Set aside.

In a large mixing bowl, add egg whites, brown sugar, yogurt, and vanilla. With a wire whisk, stir until blended, about 1 minute. Add dry ingredients to bowl. With a large rubber spatula, stir and fold until dry ingredients are just moistened. This will take about 20–25 seconds. Do not overmix. This is not a smooth batter like that of normal cakes.

Pour batter into prepared pan and bake for 35 minutes, or until toothpick inserted into the center comes out clean.

Cool in pan on a wire rack for 15 minutes. With a knife, loosen cake from sides of pan and release pan bottom from outer ring. Remove outer ring. Cool cake completely.

**Topping**

Combine cocoa and powdered sugar in a small bowl. Put cocoa mixture in a fine sieve (or sifter) and dust top of cake before serving.

*10 slices*
*Calories per slice: 188 total; 4 fat; 0 sat-fat*

## DON MAUER'S FANTASTIC FUDGE FROSTING

Frosting generally contributes a huge amount of fat to any cake. But this wonderful low-low-fat frosting does not.

¼ cup Promise Ultra Fat Free
    Margarine
6 tablespoons Dutch-process
    unsweetened cocoa powder

1 tablespoon skim milk*
¾ teaspoon vanilla extract
1¾ cup sifted powdered sugar

In a small bowl, using an electric mixer, beat margarine and cocoa on medium speed until mixture is well combined (it will appear dry and crumbly).

Turn off mixer. Add milk and vanilla to bowl. Set mixer on medium-low and mix until combined (mixture will appear thick, like clay).

Add sugar in three parts, beating after each addition. The frosting will thicken and become spreadable as you continue adding sugar. Mix until smooth and creamy and spread on cooled cake.

*1 cup frosting (approximately) — enough to ice a cake baked in*
    *an 8-inch springform pan or a two-layer 8-inch cake*
*Calories per cup: 817 total; 50 fat; 0 sat-fat*
*Calories for frosting per slice of cake\*\**

---

*To make mocha frosting, replace skim milk with brewed coffee.
\*\*If you use a cup of frosting, you can determine fat calories for the frosting on each slice of cake by dividing 50 fat calories by the number of slices of cake. To determine the total calories for frosting on each slice of cake, divide 817 total calories by the number of slices of cake.

# CHOCOLATEY-CHOCOLATE COCOA CAKE

3 tablespoons unsweetened
  cocoa
¼ cup applesauce
1 cup boiling water
1 cup sugar
1 teaspoon vanilla

1 egg yolk
1 teaspoon baking soda
½ cup buttermilk
2 cups unbleached white flour
1 teaspoon baking powder
2 egg whites

Preheat oven to 350°F. Grease a 10-inch tube pan with margarine and dust with flour.

Place cocoa and applesauce in a large mixing bowl and add boiling water.

Stir in sugar and vanilla and beat until smooth.

Stir in egg yolk and beat until smooth.

Stir baking soda into buttermilk. Add to batter and mix well.

Add flour and baking powder and mix well.

Whip egg whites until stiff but not dry and fold into batter.

Pour batter into pan and bake on middle rack of oven for 30–50 minutes or until a cake tester comes out clean.

Cool. Then frost with Don Mauer's Fantastic Fudge Frosting (page 262).

*10 slices*

| *Calories per slice:* | *Total* | *Fat* | *Sat-fat* |
| --- | --- | --- | --- |
| | 180 | 7 | 2 |
| With Fantastic Fudge Frosting | 262 | 12 | 2 |

## CINNAMON SUGAR COFFEE CAKE

This coffee cake is moist and delicious.

| | |
|---|---|
| 1½ cups unbleached white flour | 1 teaspoon cinnamon |
| 1½ teaspoons baking powder | ½ cup applesauce |
| 1 teaspoon baking soda | 1 egg |
| ½ teaspoon salt | 1 egg white |
| ¼ cup brown sugar | 1 teaspoon vanilla |
| ¾ cup sugar | 1 cup nonfat yogurt |

Preheat oven to 350°F. Grease an 8-inch springform pan with margarine.

Combine flour, baking powder, baking soda, and salt in a bowl. Set aside.

In small bowl combine ¼ cup brown sugar, ¼ cup of the granulated sugar, and cinnamon and set aside.

In a large mixing bowl, mix remaining ½ cup sugar with applesauce.

Add egg and egg white and vanilla and mix until batter is smooth.

Add flour and yogurt alternately and mix until batter is smooth.

Pour batter into springform pan.

Pour sugar mixture on top of batter and, with a knife, swirl sugar into batter.

Bake for 35–50 minutes or until cake tester comes out clean.

*8 slices*
*Calories per slice: 210 total; 7 fat; 2 sat-fat*

# CINNAMON SWEET CAKES

A family favorite that can be made on the spur of the moment.

¼ cup applesauce
1 egg
½ cup skim milk
½ cup sugar

¾ cup whole-wheat flour
¾ cup unbleached white flour
2 teaspoons baking powder
½ teaspoon salt

### Topping

½ cup brown sugar
⅓ cup coarsely chopped walnuts
1 tablespoon unbleached white
  flour

1 teaspoon cinnamon
1 tablespoon margarine

Preheat oven to 375°F. Grease an 8×8-inch baking pan with margarine.

In a large mixing bowl, beat together applesauce, egg, and skim milk.

Add sugar, whole-wheat flour, white flour, baking powder, and salt and beat until smooth.

Spoon batter into baking pan. (Batter will be thick.)

To make topping, combine brown sugar, walnuts, flour, and cinnamon in a small bowl.

Melt margarine and stir into mixture.

Sprinkle topping over batter.

Bake for about 25 minutes or until a cake tester comes out clean.

*16 squares*
*Calories per square: 120 total; 20 fat; 3 sat-fat*

## COCOA ANGEL FOOD CAKE

¾ cup cake flour                          1 teaspoon cream of tartar
¼ cup unsweetened cocoa                   1 teaspoon vanilla
1¼ cups sugar                             ½ teaspoon almond extract
1¼–1½ cups egg whites (about
    10–12)

Preheat oven to 350°F.

Sift together three times: cake flour, cocoa, and ¼ cup of the sugar. Set aside.

Sift remaining 1 cup sugar and set aside.

Whip egg whites until foamy. Add cream of tartar. Continue beating until whites are stiff but not dry.

Fold in sugar a little at a time.

Fold in vanilla and almond extract.

Sift flour-cocoa mixture over batter (one-fourth at a time) and fold into batter.

Pour batter into an ungreased 10-inch tube pan and bake for 45 minutes or until a cake tester comes out clean.

Invert tube pan and let cake cool.

*12 slices*
*Calories per slice: 119 total; <2 fat; 0 sat-fat*

# GINGER CAKE WITH PEAR SAUCE

Ginger Cake tastes good with or without pear sauce.

⅓ cup applesauce
2 tablespoons maple syrup
⅓ cup sugar
1 egg
1½ cups unbleached white flour
½ teaspoon baking powder
½ teaspoon baking soda

½ teaspoon salt
1 teaspoon cinnamon
1½ teaspoons ginger
½ teaspoon allspice
¼ teaspoon grated nutmeg
1 cup buttermilk

### Pear Sauce

2 cups water
¼ cup + 1 tablespoon sugar

3 ripe pears, peeled, cored, and
    quartered

**The Cake**

Preheat oven to 350°F. Grease an 8×8-inch baking pan with margarine.

Mix applesauce, maple syrup, and sugar until smooth.

Mix in egg.

Combine flour, baking powder, baking soda, salt, cinnamon, ginger, allspice, and nutmeg. Add to batter, alternating with buttermilk. Mix until smooth. Pour batter into baking pan and bake for 30 minutes or until a cake tester comes out clean.

Meanwhile, make pear sauce.

**The Sauce**

In a large saucepan, combine water and ¼ cup sugar and bring to a simmer.

Poach pears in sugar water for about 10 minutes or until soft.

Drain pears and purée with 1 tablespoon sugar in a blender.

Serve over cooled cake.

*16 squares*

| Calories | Total | Fat | Sat-fat |
|---|---|---|---|
| Per square | 73 | 3 | 1 |
| with Pear Sauce | 84 | 3 | 1 |

# LEMON LOAF

½ cup sugar
½ cup applesauce
Grated rind of 1 lemon
2 cups unbleached white flour
¼ teaspoon salt
2 teaspoons baking powder

1 teaspoon baking soda
¾ cup buttermilk
¼ cup fresh lemon juice
2 tablespoons fresh lemon juice
3 tablespoons sugar

Preheat oven to 375°F. Grease a loaf pan with margarine.

Mix together flour, salt, baking powder, and baking soda and set aside.

Mix buttermilk and ¼ cup lemon juice and set aside.

In a large mixing bowl, mix ½ cup sugar and applesauce.

Add grated lemon peel and mix until smooth.

Add flour mixture to applesauce mixture alternately with buttermilk mixture. *Do not overmix.*

Pour into loaf pan and bake for 30–45 minutes or until a cake tester comes out clean.

Let cool in pan 10 minutes.

In a small saucepan, combine 2 tablespoons lemon juice and 3 tablespoons sugar and stir over low heat until sugar dissolves.

Pierce top of cake with fork or skewer. Spoon lemon-sugar mixture into holes.

Let cool for easy slicing. (A whiff of lemon loaf may cause your impatient family to force you to slice the cake warm!)

*10 slices*
*Calories per slice: 150 total; 1 fat; 0 sat-fat*

# ORANGE CAKE

| | |
|---|---|
| 1½ cups unbleached white flour | ½ cup sugar |
| 2 teaspoons baking powder | ½ cup orange juice |
| ¼ teaspoon salt | 3 egg whites |
| ½ cup applesauce | 2 tablespoons orange juice |

Preheat oven to 350°F. Grease a loaf pan with margarine.

Combine flour, baking powder, and salt. Set aside.

In a large mixing bowl, beat applesauce and sugar.

Add flour mixture, alternating with ½ cup orange juice, until batter is smooth.

In another bowl, whip egg whites until stiff but not dry.

Fold egg whites into batter.

Pour batter into loaf pan and bake for 40–50 minutes or until a cake tester comes out clean.

Cool in pan for 10 minutes.

Poke holes in top of cake. Pour 2 tablespoons orange juice into holes.

*10 slices*
*Calories per slice: 119 total; 2 fat; 0 sat-fat*

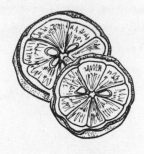

## PEACH SOUR CREAM CAKE

3 peaches
1 teaspoon sugar
2 cups cake flour
1 teaspoon baking powder
1 teaspoon baking soda
¼ teaspoon salt

½ cup applesauce
⅔ cup sugar
1 egg + 1 egg white
½ teaspoon vanilla
¼ teaspoon almond extract
1 cup nonfat sour cream

Preheat oven to 350°F. Grease an 8-inch springform pan with margarine or cooking spray.

Prepare peaches by dropping into a pot of boiling water to cover. After about 1–2 minutes, remove a peach, run under cold water, and peel. Follow the same procedure for the other peaches.

Halve each peach, take out pit, and slice thinly. Mix with 1 teaspoon sugar and set aside.

In a bowl, combine flour, baking powder, baking soda, and salt. Set aside.

Using an electric mixer, mix applesauce and sugar.

Add egg and egg white and mix until smooth.

Add vanilla and almond extract and mix until smooth.

Beating on low speed, add sour cream and flour mixture alternately and mix until just combined. Don't overmix.

Pour batter into springform pan.

Place peach slices evenly on batter to cover entire surface.

Bake for 45–50 minutes or until a cake tester comes out clean.

Remove rim and let cake cool.

*10 slices*
*Calories per slice: 174 total; 5 fat; 2 sat-fat*

# PINEAPPLE POUND CAKE

2½ cups flour
1½ teaspoons baking soda
½ teaspoon salt
1 can (8 oz.) pineapple chunks
½ cup applesauce
¾ cup sugar

3 egg whites
1 tablespoon grated orange peel
1 teaspoon vanilla
1 cup nonfat yogurt
¼ cup sugar

Preheat oven to 375°F. Grease a 10-inch tube pan with margarine.

Mix flour, baking soda, and salt and set aside.

Drain syrup from can of pineapple, reserving ¼ cup.

Mix applesauce and ¾ cup sugar.

Add egg whites, orange peel, and vanilla and beat well.

Add flour mixture and yogurt alternately to sugar mixture and mix well.

Pour half of batter into pan. Spread 1 cup (or more) of pineapple evenly over batter. Cover with remaining batter.

Bake for 40 minutes or until a cake tester comes out clean.

Let cake cool for 5 minutes.

Meanwhile, in a small saucepan, combine ¼ cup sugar with reserved pineapple syrup.

Bring to a boil, reduce heat, and simmer for 2–3 minutes or until syrup thickens slightly.

Remove cake from pan. Pierce it with a fork or skewer and spoon pineapple syrup into holes and over top of cake.

*12 slices*
*Calories per slice: 178 total; 1 fat; 0 sat-fat*

# PUMPKIN CAKE

| | |
|---|---|
| 1¼ cups unbleached white flour | ½ cup raisins |
| ½ cup rye flour | 1 cup pumpkin purée |
| 1 teaspoon baking soda | ¾ cup brown sugar |
| 1 teaspoon baking powder | 6 tablespoons margarine |
| ½ teaspoon salt | ¼ cup skim milk |
| 1½ teaspoons cinnamon | 1 egg |
| 1 teaspoon cardamom | 1 egg white |

Preheat oven to 350°F. Grease a loaf pan with margarine and lightly flour.

Combine flours, baking soda, baking powder, salt, cinnamon, cardamom, and raisins. Set aside.

In a large mixing bowl, mix together pumpkin purée, brown sugar, and margarine. Add skim milk, egg, and egg white and mix until smooth.

Stir in flour mixture.

Pour batter into loaf pan and bake for 45–60 minutes or until a cake tester comes out clean.

*18 half-inch slices*
*Calories per slice: 128 total; 34 fat; 7 sat-fat*

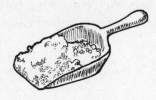

# PHILIP WAGENAAR'S
# RAISIN-GINGER-ORANGE CAKE

This is cake disguised as a quick bread. It is a sweet blending of textures and flavors. We are fortunate that Dr. Wagenaar occasionally takes time off from his biking expeditions around the world to bake.

1¾ cups unbleached white flour
2 teaspoons baking powder
½ teaspoon baking soda
½ teaspoon salt
⅓ cup applesauce
¾ cup sugar
1 tablespoon grated orange
   peel*

1 tablespoon grated lemon peel*
4 egg whites
½ cup skim milk
½ teaspoon orange extract
2 tablespoons diced crystallized
   ginger**
2 cups raisins

Preheat oven to 350°F and lightly grease a loaf pan.

Combine flour, baking powder, baking soda, and salt. Set aside.

Mix applesauce, sugar, and orange and lemon peels.

Add egg whites, two at a time, beating well after each addition.

Combine milk and orange extract.

Add milk and flour mixtures alternately to batter and beat just to mix.

Stir in ginger and raisins.

Pour batter into loaf pan and bake for 45–60 minutes or until cake tester comes out clean.

*12 slices*
*Calories per slice: 200 total; 1 fat; 0 sat-fat*

---

*A dandy way to grate orange or lemon peel is to use a zester. Or chop a few slices of it in a mini-chopper. Be sure to wash the fruit thoroughly before you remove the peel.
**Available in the spice section of most supermarkets.

# SPICE CAKE

2⅓ cups cake flour
1½ teaspoons baking powder
½ teaspoon baking soda
1 teaspoon grated nutmeg
1 teaspoon cinnamon
½ teaspoon cloves
½ teaspoon salt

¾ cup applesauce
1 cup sugar
1 egg yolk
1 cup less 2 tablespoons
   buttermilk
3 egg whites

Preheat oven to 350°F and grease a 10-inch tube pan with margarine.

Mix together flour, baking powder, baking soda, nutmeg, cinnamon, cloves, and salt and set aside.

In a large mixing bowl, mix applesauce and sugar.

Mix in egg yolk.

Add dry mixture alternately with buttermilk.

Whip 3 egg whites until stiff but not dry and fold into batter.

Pour batter into prepared pan and bake for 40–60 minutes or until cake tester comes out clean.

Cool and ice with Fantastic Fudge Frosting (page 262).

*12 slices*

| Calories per slice: | Total | Fat | Sat-fat |
|---|---|---|---|
| | 167 | 4 | 0 |
| With Fantastic Fudge Frosting | 235 | 8 | 0 |

# DEEP-DISH PEAR PIE

This pie is absolutely scrumptious! Your fortunate guests will never suspect that nonfat yogurt was substituted for the traditional sour cream (434 fat calories per cup).

Partially baked 9-inch sweet pie crust (page 276)

### Filling

2 tablespoons unbleached white
    flour
½ cup sugar
⅛ teaspoon salt
1 cup nonfat yogurt

1 egg
¼ teaspoon grated nutmeg
1 teaspoon vanilla
5 cups peeled pears (or apples),
    cut into bite-size pieces

### Topping

3 tablespoons sugar
3 tablespoons unbleached white
    flour

½ teaspoon cinnamon
4 teaspoons margarine

Preheat oven to 400°F.

In a large bowl, combine flour, sugar, and salt. Mix in nonfat yogurt. Blend in egg. Add nutmeg and vanilla. Fold in pears.

Pour pear mixture into pie crust and bake at 400°F for 15 minutes.

Lower heat to 350°F and bake for 25 minutes more.

Meanwhile, mix together topping ingredients.

Remove pie from oven and sprinkle topping over filling.

Raise heat to 375°F and bake until topping is melted — about 5–10 minutes.

*12 slices*
*Calories per slice: 215 total; 43 fat; 8 sat-fat*

# PIE, TART, OR QUICHE CRUST

1 ice cube
⅓–½ cup cold water
1⅓ cups unbleached white
   flour
2 tablespoons sugar
Pinch of salt

3 tablespoons tub margarine,
   frozen
½ tablespoon olive oil
(For nonsweet pie dough,
   eliminate sugar and add ¾
   teaspoon salt)

Place ice cube in cold water. Set aside.

Place flour in food processor fitted with steel blade or in a mixing bowl.

Add sugar and salt and mix until well blended.

Cut margarine into ½-inch pieces and add to flour mixture.

Process briefly or use pastry blender until flour mixture resembles coarse meal or oatmeal flakes.

Add oil and ⅓ cup ice water (without ice cube).

Process 2–3 seconds or blend until dough begins to collect into a ball. *Do not overprocess.*

If dough is too dry, carefully add a few more drops of cold water and blend briefly.

Remove ball of dough, lightly flour, and wrap in wax paper. Place in a plastic bag and chill in refrigerator for at least 2 hours. (Dough will keep 2–3 days in refrigerator or for several months in freezer.)

## To Bake

Preheat oven to 450°F. Grease an 8- or 9-inch pie or quiche pan with margarine.

On a piece of wax paper, roll dough into a ⅛-inch-thick circle slightly larger than pie pan.

Turn wax paper over so dough is facing downward and lay it over the pan. Peel wax paper off dough.

Gently push dough to conform to shape of pan.

Trim excess dough, except for about ¼ inch above rim of pan. Form a ridge.

Spread margarine on a piece of aluminum foil larger than the pan.

Set foil, greased-side down, on pie dough.

Fill foil with dried beans or aluminum pie weights to keep crust from bubbling up.

Bake for 7–8 minutes.

Remove foil and beans. Prick crust with a fork to release air bubbles.

For partially baked pie crust, bake 3–4 minutes more or until crust is just beginning to brown and shrink from edges of pan.

For fully baked pie crust, bake 7–10 minutes more or until lightly browned.

### One 9-inch pie crust

| Calories | Total | Fat | Sat-fat |
|---|---|---|---|
| Sweet pie crust | 1051 | 344 | 62 |
| Nonsweet pie crust | 961 | 344 | 62 |

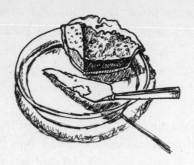

# KEY LIME PIE

This pie is as pretty to look at as it is delightful to eat. It never fails to wow guests and please the most discriminating palate. Many Key lime pies call for 3 egg yolks and butter. You will use only 1 egg yolk and margarine to create this divine dessert. You can use lemon juice instead of lime juice and call this Lemon Meringue Pie.

Partially baked 9-inch sweet pie crust (page 276) or
  Graham Cracker Crust (page 280)

### Filling

¾ cup sugar
¼ cup unbleached white flour
3 tablespoons cornstarch
¼ teaspoon salt

½–⅔ cup fresh lime juice +
  water to equal 2¼ cups
1 egg yolk
1 teaspoon margarine

### Meringue

5 egg whites, at room
  temperature

¼ teaspoon cream of tartar
½ cup + 2 tablespoons sugar

### The Filling

In a medium saucepan, thoroughly mix sugar, flour, cornstarch, and salt.

Add ¼ cup lime water and blend into a smooth paste.

Add remaining lime water and mix until smooth.

Stir filling over medium heat until it begins to boil and thicken. Remove saucepan from heat.

In a small bowl, combine egg yolk with a small amount of filling and blend until smooth. Mix back into filling in saucepan. (This step is important. If you add the egg yolk directly into the hot filling, the egg yolk will curdle.) Stir margarine into filling and pour into crust. Cool until filling gels.

### The Meringue

Preheat oven to 375°F.

Whip egg whites with cream of tartar until stiff but not dry.

Add sugar and continue beating until whites form stiff peaks.

Gently cover lime filling with egg whites, making sure they cover pie completely.

Bake for 8–10 minutes or until meringue is golden brown.

Cool at room temperature.

*10 slices*

| Calories per slice: | Total | Fat | Sat-fat |
|---|---|---|---|
| With pastry crust | 249 | 42 | 9 |
| With Graham Cracker Crust | 201 | 27 | 6 |

## GRAHAM CRACKER CRUST

Not only do Honey Graham Crackers make a delicious cookie, the crumbs make a delicious pie crust, particularly for lemon meringue or Key Lime Pie (page 278). Commercial graham crackers, graham cracker crumbs, and ready-to-bake graham cracker crusts may have more fat than you want. Make your own using the Honey Graham Crackers recipe on page 292.

8 homemade graham crackers,          1 teaspoon sugar
   crumbled (1¼ cups)                 1 tablespoon margarine

Preheat oven to 375°F.
In food processor or blender, finely crush graham crackers.
Combine crumbs and sugar and pour into pie plate.
Melt margarine and mix into crumbs.
Press crumbs into pie plate to make a crust.
Bake 8 minutes, or until lightly browned.

*One 9-inch pie crust*
*Calories per crust: 600 total; 186 fat; 34 sat-fat*

# STRAWBERRY TART

This pièce de résistance will end any meal on a high note. You can make this tart with strawberries, kiwi fruit, peaches, or most any other fruit, even lemons. Try a combination of many fruits on one tart. Tarts are typically filled with crème patissière. Instead of the egg yolks, whole milk, and butter normally used in this French custard, this strawberry tart uses packaged vanilla pudding and pie filling.

Fully baked sweet pie crust (page 276)
2 quarts strawberries
1 package vanilla pudding and pie filling
1¾ cups skim milk
1 scant tablespoon vanilla
½ cup apricot preserves
1 tablespoon sugar

Wash and hull strawberries.

On a plate the size of your tart pan, make a pleasing arrangement of strawberries.

Prepare vanilla pudding according to package instructions but use 1¾ cups skim milk and 1 scant tablespoon of vanilla instead of ingredients listed on the box.

Spread pudding evenly over bottom of pie crust.

Immediately arrange fruit on pudding.

Combine apricot preserves and sugar and heat until syrup is thick and forms a ball at end of spoon.

Paint fruit with glaze. Refrigerate tart.

*10 slices*
*Calories per slice: 194 total; 35 fat; 6 sat-fat*

## STRAWBERRY-RHUBARB PIE

The combination of rhubarb and strawberries gives this pie a wonderful blend of sweet and sour.

Partially baked sweet pie crust
  (page 276)
3 stalks rhubarb
2 pints strawberries, washed and
  hulled

1½ teaspoons margarine
¾–1 cup sugar
2⅔ tablespoons quick-cooking
  tapioca
½ teaspoon margarine

Prepare partially baked sweet pastry for pie bottom crust, but use 1¾ cups flour.

Refrigerate extra pastry.

Preheat oven to 400°F.

Slice rhubarb into ¼-inch pieces. Cut strawberries into quarters.

Gently sauté rhubarb in 1½ teaspoons of the margarine until slightly softened (about 5 minutes).

Combine rhubarb, strawberries, sugar, and tapioca, and set aside for 15 minutes.

Fill crust with fruit mixture.

Dot with remaining ½ teaspoon margarine.

Roll out remaining pastry and cut into strips. Cover pie with lattice top. Bake for 25–40 minutes or until crust is browned.

*10 slices*
*Calories per slice: 219 total; 40 fat; 7 sat-fat*

# LEMON MERINGUE ISLANDS

## Meringue Shells

4 egg whites, at room
  temperature
⅛ teaspoon salt
⅛ teaspoon cream of tartar

¾ cup sugar
½ teaspoon vanilla
¼ teaspoon almond extract

## Filling

½ cup sugar
2 tablespoons + 2 teaspoons
  flour
2 tablespoons cornstarch
⅛ tablespoon salt

⅓–½ cup fresh lemon juice +
  water to equal 1½ cups
1 egg yolk
½ teaspoon margarine

### The Meringue

Preheat oven to 275°F. Completely cover baking sheet (if it has a rim, turn baking sheet over and use the underside) with foil, dull side up. Set aside.

In a very clean mixing bowl, whip egg whites until foamy. Continue whipping as you add salt and cream of tartar. When egg whites form soft peaks, slowly add sugar. Continue to beat until whites are glossy and stiff. Fold in vanilla and almond extract.

Drop 6 large dollops of meringue evenly on foil-covered baking sheet. Use the back of a spoon or spatula to shape meringue into 6 shells, each about 4 inches across with a raised edge about ¾ inch high. Or use a pastry tube to squeeze out concentric circles to form a base and sides. The shells should be deep enough to hold the lemon custard.

Bake shells for 1 hour or until hardened. Turn off heat. Keep oven door closed. After 1 hour, remove baking sheet from oven. Carefully peel foil from bottom of meringues.

### The Filling

In a medium saucepan, thoroughly mix sugar, flour, cornstarch, and salt.

Add ¼ cup lemon water and blend into a smooth paste.

Add remaining lemon water and mix until smooth.

Stir filling over medium heat until it begins to boil and thicken. Remove saucepan from heat.

In a small bowl, combine egg yolk with a small amount of filling and blend until smooth. Mix back into filling in saucepan. (This step prevents the creation of scrambled eggs in your filling.) Stir margarine into filling. Pour into meringues. Cool.

*6 servings*
*Calories per meringue: 202 total; 8 fat; 3 sat-fat*

# MERINGUE SHELLS WITH FRESH STRAWBERRIES AND WARM RASPBERRY SAUCE

Here's a delectable dessert that has no fat. It is extremely simple to prepare and, later, to assemble. Make sure to allow 1 to 2 hours of baking time for the meringue.

### Meringue Shells

4 egg whites at room
    temperature
⅛ teaspoon salt
⅛ teaspoon cream of tartar
¾ cup sugar
½ teaspoon vanilla
¼ teaspoon almond extract

### Filling

1 pint strawberries, washed, hulled, and halved (or use other berries or
    cut-up fruit)

### Sauce

1 package (10 oz) frozen
    raspberries
1 teaspoon cornstarch
½ teaspoon lemon juice

## The Meringue

For the meringue, follow the instructions on page 283.
Fill each shell with a mound of strawberries.

## The Raspberry Sauce

Thaw raspberries or, if you forgot to plan ahead, place pouch containing raspberries in bowl of warm water for about 2 minutes to thaw. When partially thawed, purée raspberries in a blender.

Place cornstarch in a small saucepan. Add 1 tablespoon of purée and mix with cornstarch until smooth. Stir in remaining purée and add lemon juice. Bring to a boil and simmer for 1 minute.

Spoon several tablespoons of warm sauce over each strawberry-filled shell. You may also refrigerate the sauce and serve it cold.

*6 servings*
*Calories per serving: 130 total; 0 fat; 0 sat-fat*

## GLAZED CINNAMON BUNS

| | |
|---|---|
| 1 tablespoon active dry yeast | ½ cup skim milk |
| 3 tablespoons sugar | 1 egg white |
| ½ cup warm water | ⅓ cup firmly packed brown |
| 1½ cups whole-wheat flour | sugar |
| 1½+ cups unbleached white | 2 teaspoons cinnamon |
| flour | ½ cup raisins |
| 1 teaspoon salt | 1 cup confectioners' sugar |
| 1 teaspoon cinnamon | 1–3 tablespoons skim milk |
| 1½ tablespoons olive oil | 1 teaspoon vanilla |

Place yeast, sugar, and water in a large bowl or the bowl of a food processor. Let proof until foamy.

Add whole-wheat flour, 1½ cups white flour, salt, 1 teaspoon cinnamon, oil, milk, and egg white and mix or process. Keep adding white flour until dough becomes fairly stiff.

Knead dough for 10 minutes or process for 15 seconds or until dough is smooth and elastic, adding more flour if necessary.

Place dough in a bowl greased with a drop or two of olive oil, cover with a dish towel, and let rise in a warm place for 1 hour or until doubled in bulk.

When dough has doubled in size, place it on a lightly floured surface.

Grease a 12-cup muffin tin with margarine. Set aside.

While dough rests, combine brown sugar, 2 teaspoons cinnamon, and raisins and set aside.

Roll dough into a 9×12-inch rectangle.

Sprinkle cinnamon mixture evenly over dough.

Starting with long side of rectangle, roll dough *tightly* into a jelly roll. Cut it crosswise into 12 even pieces.

Place each piece, cut side up, in a muffin cup. Cover with a towel and let rise 45 minutes.

Preheat oven to 400°F. Bake buns for 15–20 minutes or until nicely browned. Transfer to a cooling rack.

Place confectioners' sugar in bowl of an electric mixer. Add 1 table-spoon milk and vanilla and mix on low speed until smooth. Add more milk very slowly if mixture is too thick.

Spoon glaze over tops of buns.

*12 buns*
*Calories per bun: 120 total; 18 fat; 3 sat-fat*

## COCOA BROWNIES

⅓ cup margarine

½ cup sugar

¼ cup light corn syrup

2 teaspoons vanilla

1 egg

1 egg white

⅓ cup unsweetened cocoa

½ cup flour

½ teaspoon salt

½ cup chopped walnuts

Preheat oven to 350°F. Grease an 8×8-inch baking pan with margarine.

In a large bowl, cream margarine and sugar.

Add corn syrup, vanilla, egg, and egg white and mix until well blended.

Combine cocoa, flour, and salt and slowly add to batter.

Fold in nuts and pour batter into baking pan.

Bake for 25–30 minutes or until a cake tester comes out clean.

*16 squares*
*Calories per square: 115 total; 54 fat; 9 sat-fat*

# PUDDING BROWNIES

### Batter

| | |
|---|---|
| 1 cup unbleached white flour | ½ teaspoon salt |
| ½ cup sugar | ½ cup skim milk |
| ¼ cup unsweetened cocoa | ¼ cup applesauce |
| 2 teaspoons baking powder | 1 teaspoon vanilla |

### Topping

| | |
|---|---|
| 3 tablespoons unsweetened cocoa | ⅓ cup brown sugar |
| | 1 cup hot water |

### The Batter

Preheat oven to 350°F. Grease an 8×8-inch baking pan with margarine or cooking spray.

In a large mixing bowl, mix together flour, sugar, cocoa, baking powder, and salt.

Stir in milk, applesauce, and vanilla.

Spoon batter into pan.

### The Topping

In a small bowl, combine cocoa and brown sugar. Mix in hot water. Pour mixture over batter in pan.

Bake for 30 minutes or until cake tester comes out clean.

Cool brownies in pan.

Remove to serving plate. Take excess pudding from pan bottom and "ice" brownies with it.

Serve warm or refrigerate.

*16 squares*
*Calories per square: 83 total; 2 fat; 0 sat-fat*

## PUMPKIN PUDDING SOUFFLÉ

This is a cross between a pudding and a soufflé. It's a bit strange looking, but it tastes delicious.

½ cup + 2 tablespoons sugar
½ teaspoon salt
1 teaspoon cinnamon
½ teaspoon ground ginger
¼ teaspoon ground cloves
¼ teaspoon freshly ground
   nutmeg

3 egg whites
1¾ cups (15-oz can) pumpkin
1½ cups evaporated skim
   milk
Unbaked pie crust (page 276)

Preheat oven to 425°F. Grease an 8-inch springform pan with margarine or cooking spray.

Combine sugar, salt, cinnamon, ginger, cloves, and nutmeg. Set aside.

Whip egg whites until stiff but not dry. Set aside.

In a large bowl, stir sugar-spice mixture into pumpkin.

Stir milk into pumpkin until completely blended.

Fold egg whites into pumpkin until completely blended.

Pour into pan.

Bake for 15 minutes at 425°F. Lower heat to 350°F and bake for 40 or 50 minutes or until knife inserted near center comes out clean. Cool.

*10 slices*
*Calories per slice: 97 total; 2 fat; 0 sat-fat*

# COCOA MERINGUE KISSES

For a special treat, eat these delectable morsels right from the oven. Pop a whole kiss in your mouth and savor the taste of warm, melting chocolate. (But use some restraint. Altogether, they add up to a lot of empty sugar calories.)

| | |
|---|---|
| 2 egg whites | 1 teaspoon vanilla |
| ⅛ teaspoon cream of tartar | 2 tablespoons cocoa |
| ¾ cup sugar | |

Preheat oven to 325°F. Line a cookie sheet with foil, dull side up.

With an electric beater, whip egg whites and cream of tartar until foamy.

Add sugar 1 tablespoon at a time. Add vanilla. Beat until whites form stiff peaks.

Fold in cocoa.

Drop meringue onto foil by teaspoonfuls in the shape of a candy kiss.

Bake for 20 minutes. Wait for a few minutes, then slide a knife or spatula under kisses and they will lift off foil.

*32 kisses (approximately)*
*Calories per kiss: 20 total; 0 fat; 0 sat-fat*

# HONEY GRAHAM CRACKERS

| | |
|---|---|
| 1 cup whole-wheat flour | 2 tablespoons margarine |
| ½ cup unbleached white flour | 2 tablespoons light brown sugar |
| ½ teaspoon baking powder | 2 tablespoons honey |
| ¼ teaspoon baking soda | ½ teaspoon vanilla |
| Pinch of salt | 2 tablespoons skim milk |

Preheat oven to 350°F and grease a cookie sheet with margarine.

Combine flours, baking powder, baking soda, and salt and set aside.

Cream margarine, sugar, and honey in an electric mixer.

Mix in vanilla.

Add flour mixture and milk.

Gather dough together (add a drop or two of milk if too dry) and knead into a ball.

Roll dough onto cookie sheet in a rectangle, ⅛ inch thick.

If dough is too sticky, sprinkle it with flour.

Without moving dough, cut into 3-inch squares.

Lightly score a line through the center of each square and pierce each side several times with a fork.

Bake 10–15 minutes, until edges brown. Remove crackers and cool on a wire rack.

Crackers will become crisp as they cool.

*18 crackers*
*Calories per cracker: 58 total; 12 fat; 2 sat-fat*

# MANDELBROT

⅔ cup sugar
¼ cup olive oil
3 egg whites
1 egg

1½ cups unbleached white flour
1 teaspoon baking powder
½ cup coarsely ground almonds
1 teaspoon orange extract

Preheat oven to 350°F.

Lightly grease a cookie sheet with margarine or olive oil.

In a large mixing bowl, cream sugar and olive oil.

Mix in egg whites and egg.

Add flour and baking powder and mix until smooth.

Stir in almonds and orange extract.

Pour onto cookie sheet. Spread into square (8×8 inches), about ½ inch thick.

Bake for 20 minutes or until lightly browned.

Remove cookie sheet from oven.

Cut dough into strips about 3 inches wide and then score (do not cut through) into bars about ¾ inch wide.

Turn strips over and bake 10 more minutes or until crisp.

Break into bars.

*4 dozen bars*
*Calories per bar: 46 total; 18 fat; 2 sat-fat*

## COCOA OATMEAL COOKIES

These low-fat cookies are one of the many wonderful recipes found in *Delightful Dishes by Friends Against Fat,* a cookbook compiled by the participants of the first *Choose to Lose* course given by Wellness Together of Garrett County Memorial Hospital, Garrett County, Maryland. Thank you, Kendra Stemple Todd and your participants!

⅔ cup unbleached white flour

⅔ cup sugar

1 cup rolled oats

⅓ cup unsweetened cocoa

1 teaspoon baking powder

1 teaspoon baking soda

½ teaspoon salt

2 egg whites

⅓ cup corn syrup

1 teaspoon vanilla

Preheat oven to 350°F and grease a cookie sheet with margarine or a cooking spray.

In a large mixing bowl, combine flour, sugar, oats, cocoa, baking powder, baking soda, and salt.

Add egg whites, corn syrup, and vanilla. Stir just until dry ingredients are moistened.

Drop batter by teaspoonfuls onto cookie sheet and bake for 10 minutes or until set.

Cool for 5 minutes on cookie sheet. Remove immediately or cookies will harden and will be difficult to remove.

*2 dozen cookies (approximately)*
*Calories per cookie: 69 total; 5 fat; 0 sat-fat*

# SUPER OATMEAL COOKIES

These oatmeal cookies are called "super" because they are absolutely delicious and as a bonus have only 2 fat calories (from the oatmeal) each.

1 cup unbleached white flour
1 cup rolled oats (not quick-
    cooking)
½ cup sugar
½ teaspoon baking powder
½ teaspoon baking soda

½ teaspoon salt
½ teaspoon cinnamon
2 egg whites
⅓ cup light corn syrup
1 teaspoon vanilla
½ cup raisins

Preheat oven to 375°F. Grease a cookie sheet with margarine or cooking spray.

In a bowl, combine flour, oats, sugar, baking powder, baking soda, salt, and cinnamon. Mix well. Set aside.

In a large mixing bowl, beat together egg whites, corn syrup, and vanilla.

Add dry ingredients and mix until well blended. Mix in raisins. Batter will be sticky.

Drop batter by heaping teaspoonfuls about 2 inches apart onto cookie sheet.

Bake 10–15 minutes or until golden. Cool.

*24 cookies*
*Calories per cookie: 67 total; 2 fat; 0 sat-fat*

## CHEWY OATMEAL-FRUIT BARS

½ cup unbleached white flour
¼ cup whole-wheat flour
½ teaspoon baking soda
½ teaspoon ground cinnamon
¼ teaspoon salt
⅓ cup granulated sugar
⅓ cup brown sugar
½ cup mashed banana

1 tablespoon olive oil
1 egg
1 tablespoon buttermilk
1 teaspoon vanilla
1½ cups rolled oats
½ cup raisins and dried
   cranberries

Preheat oven to 350°F. Grease an 8×8-inch baking pan with margarine or cooking spray.

In a medium bowl, combine flours, baking soda, cinnamon, and salt and set aside.

In a large mixing bowl, combine sugars, banana, oil, egg, buttermilk, and vanilla and mix well.

Add flour mixture and mix well.

Add oats and dried fruit.

Spread mixture evenly over pan. Bake 20–30 minutes or until lightly browned.

Cool and cut into bars.

*12 bars*
*Calories per bar: 150 total; 20 fat; 4 sat-fat*

## SUGAR COOKIES

These cookies may be habit forming. They contain only 3 sat-fat calories each, but the 11 total fat calories per cookie can quickly add up.

3 tablespoons margarine
⅔ cup + ⅓ cup sugar
1 egg
2 teaspoons vanilla

1 tablespoon skim milk
1¾ cups + ⅓ cup unbleached white flour
½ teaspoon baking soda

Preheat oven to 350°F. Grease a cookie sheet with a bit of margarine.

In a large mixing bowl, cream margarine and ⅔ cup of the sugar.

Mix in egg, vanilla, and skim milk.

Add 1¾ cups flour and baking soda and mix until smooth.

Pour remaining ⅓ cup sugar onto a small plate. Pour remaining flour on another small plate. Dip your fingers in the flour, pick up a small amount of dough, and roll dough into a small ball in your hand.

Roll ball in sugar. Place ball on cookie sheet and gently flatten with your hand. Continue with the rest of the dough.

Bake for 10–15 minutes or until golden brown.

*32 cookies*
*Calories per cookie: 65 total; 11 fat; 2 sat-fat*

# PEARS HÉLÈNE

Pears Hélène made with cocoa and margarine are wonderful, just like their counterpart made with chocolate and butter.

The chocolate sauce is a good all-purpose dessert sauce. You can store it in the refrigerator for weeks.

### Pears

4 ripe pears
2 cups water

¼ cup sugar
1 tablespoon fresh lemon juice

### Chocolate Sauce

3 tablespoons sugar
2 tablespoons unsweetened cocoa
1 tablespoon cornstarch

2 tablespoons water
1 tablespoon light corn syrup
1 tablespoon margarine
½ teaspoon vanilla

## The Pears

Peel pears, cut in half, core, and cut off stems.

In a pot large enough to hold pears, combine water, sugar, and lemon juice and bring to a boil.

Spoon pears into liquid, reduce heat, and simmer, covered, for 5 minutes. Pears should be tender, not mushy.

Drain poached pears and chill.

## The Chocolate Sauce

In a small saucepan, combine sugar, cocoa, and cornstarch.

Mix in water and corn syrup and blend well.

Cook over medium heat until mixture comes to a boil.

Remove from heat and stir for about 1 minute.

Add margarine and vanilla and continue to stir until sauce is well blended.

Place 2 pear halves, cut-side up, on each plate, and pour warm sauce over them.

*4 servings*
*Calories per serving: 205 total; 23 fat; 5 sat-fat*

# Index

# MORE HEALTHY-EATING BOOKS BY THE GOORS:

## CHOOSE TO LOSE® A FOOD LOVER'S GUIDE TO PERMANENT WEIGHT LOSS

by Dr. Ron and Nancy Goor
Houghton Mifflin Company, Third Edition, 1999

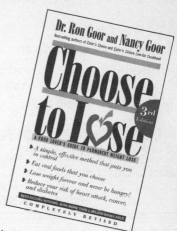

- **Eat like a normal person!**
- **Never be hungry!**
- **Lose weight permanently**

**Choose to Lose** is different. You never starve because you *have* to eat a lot of food — of course, low-fat, nutritious food. You are never deprived because you can fit in high-fat favorites. You are empowered to make wise choices in every situation. You are in control. You will feel GREAT about yourself.

**AND IT WORKS!** Barbara L., Bronx, New York, who lost 85 pounds, writes, "I still have all the weight off and that is after 9 years! Everyone I know keeps asking me how I have kept it off and I just say, read **Choose to Lose** and you will find out."

## EATER'S CHOICE
## A FOOD LOVER'S GUIDE TO LOWER CHOLESTEROL

by Dr. Ron and Nancy Goor
Houghton Mifflin Company, Fifth Edition, 1999

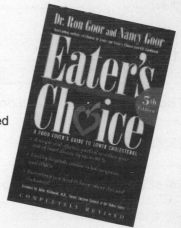

- Everything you need to know about diet, cholesterol, and heart disease, including updated information on trans fats, reversal of coronary heart disease, cholesterol-lowering drugs, etc.
- A simple method to reduce your risk of heart disease by up to 60 percent
- Chapter on children and cholesterol

**Both books are available at most bookstores or use order form on next page.**

**Visit our website: http://www.choicediets.com**

# Books on healthy eating by Dr. Ron and Nancy Goor

## CHOOSE TO LOSE
### A Food Lover's Guide to Permanent Weight Loss

If you need to lose weight, *Choose to Lose: A Food Lover's Guide to Permanent Weight Loss* will show you how. It's easy and nonpunishing. (see preceding page)

## EATER'S CHOICE
### A Food Lover's Guide to Lower Cholesterol

Everything you need to know about diet, cholesterol, and heart disease and an easy method to lower your cholesterol up to 33% and risk of heart disease up to 66%. (see preceding page)

## EATER'S CHOICE LOW-FAT COOKBOOK

320 delicious, easy-to-make, low-fat recipes for family, friends, and company. Makes following *Eater's Choice* a piece of cake. (see preceding page)

**Visit our website: http://www.choicediets.com**

**TO ORDER:** For quickest delivery: call toll-free 1-888-897-9360 and order by credit card. Or fill out and send order form below with check or money order payable to Choice Diets, Inc.

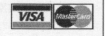

---

**SHIP TO:** Print clearly or type  **ORDER FORM**

Name _____

Address _____

City _____ State _____ Zip _____

| ITEM | QUANTITY | PRICE EACH | TOTAL PRICE | |
|---|---|---|---|---|
| **Choose to Lose** (3rd edition) | | $17.00 | | |
| **Eater's Choice** (5th edition) | | 17.00 | | |
| **Eater's Choice Low-Fat Cookbook** | | 16.00 | | |
| Send check or money order to: | 5% tax (MD residents) | | | |
| **Choice Diets, Inc.**<br>**P.O. Box 2053**<br>**Rockville, MD 20847-2053** | Postage and Handling | | 2 | 00 |
| | **TOTAL ORDER** | $ | | |

Call toll-free 1-888-897-9360 to see if a
Choose to Lose Weight Loss/Healthy Eating Program is near you.

Prices are subject to change.